Praise for...

Miller's Review of Critical Vaccine Studies:
400 Important Scientific Papers Summarized for Parents and Researchers

"*Miller's Review of Critical Vaccine Studies* confirms that the truth is stubborn and eventually wins out. In the worldwide and U.S. debate between fact-based vaccine science and pharmaceutical, political, and media driven pseudoscience, we now have a powerful document that makes it clear to any parent or sincere scientist that vaccines are not only inadequate and unsafe but actively disrupt normal immune, neurological, and brain development. Vaccines increased rates of acute and chronic diseases, allergies, asthma, seizures, attention deficit disorder, autoimmune ailments, type 1 diabetes, autism, hospitalizations, sudden infant death, and a variety of other adverse health conditions. With these facts, it is no wonder that the U.S., which has the highest vaccine requirements, has the highest amount of sick and chronically ill children in the industrialized world. In addition, this book summarizes research on the ecology of microorganisms showing them being altered by vaccines toward a more health-endangering outcome. The phenomenon of 'strain replacement' has created more virulent and vaccine-resistant pathogens (similar to antibiotic resistant bacteria and tuberculosis, which are causing fatalities). This book is so precise and exciting in addressing the vaccine controversy that I read it in one evening. Neil Miller did an extraordinarily masterful job in gathering these vaccine facts, highlighting the moral and ethical issues that are being raised. I recommend this book to any parent who has questions about vaccines and wants to be factually educated to make informed decisions."

—*Rabbi Gabriel Cousens, MD, MD(H), DD*

"Researcher and author, Neil Miller, scoured and summarized published studies on vaccines for you, the reader. Nowhere else can one find such an organized and concise compilation of research on vaccines. Not only does Miller have a deep understanding of science and the issues at hand, he has made this book easy to reference and cite. Truly, there is no other guide out there quite like it. For everyone who contacts me in the future seeking scientific evidence about vaccines, I will recommend *Miller's Review of Critical Vaccine Studies*."

—*Toni Bark, MD, MHEM, LEED AP, previous Director of the pediatric ER at Michael Reese Hospital*

"Neil Miller's book is a tour de force and a clarion voice championing the cautionary principle: '*When in doubt, minimize risk.*' Tragically, this is a wisdom entirely lost on our elected representatives due to the persuasive lobbyists of Big Pharma. In these pages, you have powerful and unambiguous data which exposes the myriad problems with vaccinations, as well as with government officials who force these unproven and dangerous injections into vulnerable defenseless infants — and soon, if recent legislation is not reversed, into all American citizens. Many scientists alive today know that something is, indeed, rotten in the state of our medical industrial complex. We scientists and scientifically-oriented medical doctors rely upon peer-reviewed scientific literature, but too often that treasure trove is compromised by blatant conflicts of interest. Now, Mr. Miller has studiously sifted through the literature and revealed the truth of the matter. At present, criticisms leveled against opponents of vaccinations are insubstantial ad hominem personal attacks. Let's talk science. Read this book. The truth will keep you and your children protected."

—*Bradford S. Weeks, MD*

"If you trust vaccines to protect you without harm, then you need to read this book. Miller provides a multitude of peer-reviewed scientific articles showing the gaping chinks in the alleged 'vaccines are safe and effective' dogma. If, after having read the information herein, you still believe vaccines should be forcibly administered to all children, or that you should blindly consent to all vaccines recommended for adults, your decision will forever remain a mystery to me."

—Robert Jay Rowen, MD, Founder of Medical Freedom in USA, former member of Alaska State Medical Board, Board Eligible (Previously Certified) in Family and Emergency Medicine

"When I graduated from medical school, the Dean told my class, 'We have just taught you the most up-to-date medical information. Unfortunately, at least 50% of what we taught you was wrong. It is your job to go out in the world and figure out which part was right and which was wrong.' I think the Dean may have underestimated the wrong part. *Miller's Review of Critical Vaccine Studies* shatters the often-repeated statement that 'vaccines are safe and effective for everyone.' This book should be required reading for every doctor, medical student and parent. Reading this book will allow you to make better choices when considering vaccination."

—David Brownstein, MD, Medical Director, Center for Holistic Medicine, West Bloomfield, MI

"In medical school, we are trained that vaccines are safe and effective and to ignore adverse reactions listed in the manufacturers' vaccine inserts since it is just jargon from lawyers. Then we are given the vaccine schedule to implement and we have our patients read a one-page form that minimizes any risk so we can call this informed consent. Neil Miller's book gives a great review of studies showing the other side. In order to give proper informed consent, we must know the benefits *and risks*. I hope that with the awareness of actual risks, in which we are just at the tip of the iceberg thanks to cognitive dissonance, we can at least better risk-stratify our most vulnerable patients so we can decrease collateral damage while trying to satisfy the desire to 'protect the greater good.'"

—Cammy Benton, MD, ABIHM

"Although all published studies must be carefully examined for reliability, *Miller's Review* offers a significant sample (n = 400) of investigations likely to crack the blissful consensus of governmental agencies concerning the supposed benefits of 'immunization' considered as a *whole* (rather than as a series of distinct pharmaceutical products requiring complex *individual* assessments to objectively determine their benefits, hazards and cost). Vaccines are promoted as an all-out offensive, mainly for the greatest advantage of the manufacturers and their professional obligees: agency experts, academics, and health professionals in their majority."

—Marc Girard, MD, MSc, independent consultant for the pharmaceutical industry

"This is a well-researched work that raises a number of important considerations about our current vaccination practices. Through studies with commentaries, the reader is led on a journey that bypasses the typical myopic view our society has toward vaccines."

—Brandon Horn, PhD, JD, LAc, Chief Academic Officer, American University of Complementary Medicine

"*Miller's Review of Critical Vaccine Studies* is the most comprehensive and coherent accumulation of peer-reviewed research on vaccine issues and natural immunity I have ever come across. A must read for parents, teachers, doctors and other healthcare providers."

—Dr. Tyson Perez, pediatric chiropractor

Miller's Review of Critical Vaccine Studies

400 Important Scientific Papers Summarized for Parents and Researchers

Neil Z. Miller

New Atlantean Press
Santa Fe, New Mexico

Miller's Review of Critical Vaccine Studies

400 Important Scientific Papers Summarized for Parents and Researchers

by Neil Z. Miller

ISBN: 978-188121740-4

Library of Congress Cataloging-in-Publication Data

Miller, Neil Z., author.
Miller's review of critical vaccine studies : 400 important scientific papers summarized for parents and researchers / Neil Z. Miller.
p. ; cm.
Review of critical vaccine studies
Includes bibliographical references and index.
ISBN 978-1-881217-40-4
I. Title. II. Title: Review of critical vaccine studies.
[DNLM: 1. Vaccination. 2. Vaccines. 3. Biomedical Research. 4. Child. 5. Safety. QW 805]
RA638
614.4'7--dc23
2015025036

Cover photo: Bigstock

Printed in the United States of America

Published by:
New Atlantean Press
PO Box 9638
Santa Fe, NM 87504
www.new-atlantean.com

This publication is dedicated
to parents and their children.

Warning/Disclaimer/Disclosure

- The information in this book — *Miller's Review of Critical Vaccine Studies* — is for educational and informational purposes only, and is not intended to be a substitute for medical care and advice. Licensed health practitioners are available for that purpose.

- The author has endeavored to accurately summarize scientific papers that are critical of vaccines. However, errors can occur. Therefore, readers are urged to verify all of the data and references in this book.

- Some of the information presented in this book may conflict with data presented elsewhere. Therefore, readers are encouraged to seek professional guidance in evaluating contradictory, complex or confusing information. If you are pregnant or have other special conditions requiring medical attention, consult with your physician.

- *Miller's Review of Critical Vaccine Studies* is not endorsed by vaccine manufacturers, the American Academy of Pediatrics, the FDA, CDC or any other federal, state or "official" organization. For official information about vaccines, contact vaccine manufacturers, the FDA, CDC and World Health Organization.

- Vaccine recommendations change rapidly. Immunization schedules are periodically revised. Therefore, the FDA and CDC should be consulted for the most up-to-date information regarding who should or should not receive vaccines, at what ages, and the number of doses.

- *Miller's Review* does not recommend for or against vaccines. Parents and other concerned people are responsible for making those decisions. The information in this book tends to find faults with vaccines, therefore readers are advised to balance the data presented here with data presented by "official" sources of vaccine information, including vaccine manufacturers, the FDA, CDC and World Health Organization.

- Any headline or statement in this book claiming that a vaccine *caused* an unwelcome event indicates that it preceded the event and there is scientific evidence of its actual or contributing influence. Read the original paper for clarification of the authors' findings. The information in this book was composed in accordance with best fair use practices.

- This book is sold with the understanding that the author and publisher are not providing medical, legal or other professional advice. The author and publisher do not recommend for or against vaccines. All of the information in this book is taken from other sources and includes original citations. If you have questions, doubts, or concerns regarding any of the data in this book, go to the original source or consult with your doctor. Then research this topic even further so that you may make wise and informed vaccine decisions.

Contents

Foreword

Gary Goldman, PhD

In modern times, unprecedented advances in the medical field — such as knee and hip replacements — have improved our quality of life. Emergency medical procedures have saved countless lives by restoring damaged or injured organs and tissues. When my three children were young, I believed that vaccines were a medical marvel as well, and they received their full complement of vaccines as prescribed by their physician according to the recommended vaccination schedule. So, when I was hired by the Los Angeles County Department of Health Services *(Acute Communicable Disease Control Unit)*, to help conduct epidemiological studies of varicella disease in the local community known as Antelope Valley (which consisted of approximately 300,000 residences principally in Palmdale and Lancaster, California), I was thrilled to participate. I would be working at one of three active surveillance sites funded by the Centers for Disease Control and Prevention (CDC) to study the impact of the newly recommended chickenpox vaccine, which was just being introduced into the U.S. child population. It was 1995, and with enthusiasm I reflected on the prospect that data from this research project would not only be helpful to the community in which my family and I resided, but also provide insight into how the CDC formulates national policies in connection with the chickenpox vaccine.

I served as an Epidemiology Analyst. All positive results and trends that I reported were quickly reviewed and subsequently published in medical journal articles whose authorship honored CDC officials, physicians serving as the co-principal investigators, the project director, myself, and the data collection assistants. By the end of five years, after widespread varicella vaccination, our data demonstrated an 80% decline in varicella disease in the community. In addition, the chickenpox vaccine appeared to be safe. My performance reviews were outstanding and I was encouraged to contribute additional investigations that might lead to further publications.

By the end of 1999, long-term nurses in local schools were reporting cases of shingles (herpes zoster) occurring among children where previously such case reports had been extremely rare. Based on this observation, I recommended that shingles be added to our active surveillance project. The shingles case reports should have been collected from the start of the project since both chickenpox and shingles are caused by the same varicella zoster virus. After experiencing a case of chickenpox, the virus remains dormant until the body's cell-mediated immunity declines to a certain low level at which point the varicella zoster virus can reactivate as shingles. Each time an adult is exposed to a child having chickenpox, the adult receives an exogenous (external) immune boost that helps suppress or postpone the onset of shingles, thus serving as a free and valuable benefit to the adult that could yield a protective effect lasting many years.

My observation of a relationship between chickenpox and shingles was not new. In 1965, Dr. Hope-Simpson, serving as a physician in Cirencester, England, studied herpes zoster among the local population. [*Proc R Soc Med* 1965; 58: 9-20.] He was the first to propose the hypothesis that the rates, or incidence, of shingles in each age group were perhaps due to that group's exposure to cases of chickenpox. Using approximate incidence rates, the rate of shingles among children aged 1 to 10 years and among adolescents aged 11 to 19 years were the lowest, because so many in these age groups contracted chickenpox and had frequent re-exposure to the disease. During adulthood, the incidence of shingles quadrupled by age 50, due to older adults' diminishing exposure to children with chickenpox. Thus, while shingles was primarily thought of as increasing with the onset of old age, in reality, shingles increased as adults experienced fewer contacts with children infected with chickenpox, which in turn caused a decrease in subclinical boosting. In a study of physicians who had frequent contact with children, findings demonstrated that the rate of shingles was one-fourth to one-eighth that of other adults in the same age-group in the general population that typically had less frequent exposure. [*Kansenshokagu Zasshi* 1995; 69(8): 908-12.]

After collecting two years of shingles case reports in the community, I observed that the incidence of shingles among unvaccinated children who had previously contracted chickenpox was unusually high, approaching the rate seen in adults. This was a foreboding result indicating that universal varicella vaccination could have the effect of increasing the incidence of shingles for a period of 50 or more years among adults who had a prior case of chickenpox — usually a benign case in their youth. Since about 25% of medical costs associated with the varicella zoster virus are due to varicella and about 75% are due to shingles, any increase in shingles would easily offset any cost benefit associated with a reduction in cases of chickenpox.

The CDC had justified its recommendation that all U.S. children receive a chickenpox vaccine based on the cost savings to society attributed to parents not having to stay home from work to care for their child with chickenpox. Further initial cost/benefit assumptions that justified varicella vaccination included, 1) a vaccine cost of $35, 2) one vaccine offering lifetime protection, and 3) no deleterious effects on the closely related shingles epidemiology. These assumptions all proved to be invalid. The current vaccine cost is approximately $100, a two-dose vaccination policy was instituted due to the occurrence of breakthrough varicella disease (vaccinated children were still contracting chickenpox), and recent research on herpes zoster incidence supports Dr. Hope-Simpson's hypothesis that exposures to chickenpox have a protective effect to suppress or prevent the reactivation of shingles in adults. [*Am J Epidemiol* 2013; 77(10): 1134-42.] Instead of stopping the universal varicella vaccination of children in the U.S., the CDC added a second booster dose for children and introduced a shingles vaccine for older adults (who previously received boosts to their immunity at no charge by virtue of the annual outbreaks of chickenpox in their communities).

I prepared a paper for review and subsequent publication summarizing the first two years of shingles data. Such review was never forthcoming and I was instructed not to pursue any further investigation of shingles rates in the Antelope Valley. I did not want to become involved in research fraud, so I resigned after eight years of employment and sought to publish the other side of the research data that I felt was being suppressed. However, prior to having several papers published in the journal *Vaccine,* I received a notice from the Los Angeles County legal department to "cease and desist."

With the assistance of an experienced attorney, I overcame the CDC's objection that the data was confidential, and these studies were published. (Some of them are summarized in this book.) The CDC also improperly challenged the methodology that I used and results I derived. However, several years later they published a paper on herpes zoster using methodology similar to that specified in my papers that they had earlier criticized. The CDC presented herpes zoster incidence rates that closely compared to those I had published following my resignation. [*Vaccine* 2013 Mar 25; 31(13): 1683, Table 1.]

In marketing the varicella vaccine, the vaccine manufacturer used commercials highlighting that a child could die from chickenpox. The chance of this occurring is about the same as a child being struck by lightning. Unfortunately, vaccine research is largely financed by the pharmaceutical companies producing the vaccine or by health agencies that have conflicts of interest with these companies. (Studies that confirm such conflicts of interest are summarized in this book.) In addition, many CDC-sponsored studies, and other studies promoting vaccines, do not provide raw data to replicate the findings, which is a necessary component of science. Thus, published findings in medical journals and the positive claims associated with any given vaccine are often propaganda — one-sided promotions that fail to disclose any negative effects, which at times can be significant. For example, a recent paper by Hooker and Kern et al. found evidence of malfeasance in CDC research purporting to show that thimerosal (a mercury-based preservative added to some vaccines) is safe. Although more than 165 studies examined thimerosal and found it to be dangerous, the CDC claims that it is safe and unrelated to autism. The CDC's claim that thimerosal is safe for use in vaccines and does not cause autism is based on just six studies that it sponsored. Four of the studies withheld important results from final publication and all of them are methodologically unsound. [*BioMed Research International* 2014; article ID 247218.] These tactics produce continual cycles of disease and treatment.

Following my work with the Los Angeles County Department of Health Services and the CDC, I continued to engage in vaccine research and discovered that my experience with the varicella vaccine was only the tip of the iceberg. In fact, if my children were born today, I would not permit them to be vaccinated. Vaccines with their associated adjuvants can cause serious long-term adverse effects in the form of autoimmune disorders and other chronic detrimental health conditions. Ongoing research continues to elucidate the complexities of the human immune system, providing an improved understanding of the biological mechanisms responsible for adverse vaccine reactions. In addition, the current childhood vaccination schedule is much more crowded than previous schedules, with infants receiving several vaccines during their pediatric well-baby visits. Multiple vaccines administered concomitantly may increase the risk of death. [*PloS One* 2011 Jan 26; 6(1): e16363; *Hum Exp Toxicol* 2012; 31(10): 1012-21.]

The National Library of Medicine has a multitude of studies that warn of these negative outcomes, including the possibility of vaccine-related fatalities which can sometimes be characterized as SIDS — sudden infant death syndrome. Detailed toxicological examinations of post-mortem brains and tissues, as well as other specialized investigations, have indeed documented vaccine-related deaths. Yet, there is a movement to make vaccination compulsory, removing all current vaccine exemptions, which will effectively eliminate the doctrine of informed consent, essential for the preservation of human rights.

Rising healthcare costs are, in part, the result of biased scientific research that supports an ever-expanding list of required vaccines that, in reality, have a negative cost and health benefit. Such vaccines create a life-long stream of income flowing into the healthcare system treating all of the people who experience adverse vaccine reactions. About 30,000 reports of suspected adverse vaccine reactions are filed with the U.S. government every year and more than $3.1 billion has already been paid to compensate vaccine victims and their families.

Through independent analysis, it is possible to uncover the lies and deception emanating from the public relations propaganda produced by the vaccine manufacturers and healthcare institutions themselves. This book, *Miller's Review of Critical Vaccine Studies,* can assist the reader so that any decision to vaccinate or not is an informed one. The author, Neil Z. Miller, deserves high commendation for his boldness in providing research material in a format that can assist parents and other researchers in their investigation of vaccine truths while gaining a more circumspect understanding of tradeoffs associated with vaccine issues. This invaluable resource with its straightforward summaries of harmful effects that peer-reviewed published research on vaccines has revealed can positively impact the health and lives of millions of children, adolescents and adults.

Introduction

Many people sincerely believe that all vaccines are safe, adverse reactions are rare, and no peer-reviewed scientific studies exist showing that vaccines can cause harm. A more reasonable perspective, however, is that while vaccines may contribute toward enhancing immunity against contracting specific diseases, they also are responsible for causing autoimmune disorders and other detrimental long-term effects that are rarely disclosed. This book — *Miller's Review of Critical Vaccine Studies* — provides the other side of the story that is not commonly told. It contains summaries of more than 400 important scientific papers to help parents and researchers enhance their understanding of vaccinations.

The studies in this book do not support vaccine safety and effectiveness. Instead, they provide scientific evidence of risks and detriments, confirming adverse side effects or tradeoffs associated with vaccination. For example, the vaccine might decrease the likelihood of contracting a contagious ailment while increasing the odds of developing a neurological disorder, immunological injury, or coronary heart disease. In addition, allergies, seizures, diabetes and thrombocytopenia (a life-threatening autoimmune disease that causes internal bleeding) are more likely in vaccinated populations. Vaccinated children may also be trading a reduced risk of infections for an increased risk of cancer.

Most of the scientific papers summarized in this book are peer-reviewed studies published in medical journals indexed by the U.S. National Library of Medicine (the world's largest medical library). They include meta-analyses, systematic reviews of the scientific literature, randomized placebo-controlled studies, cohort studies, case control studies, case series, professional scientific commentary, and animal research. Nearly all of the studies provide crucial evidence of vaccine safety or immunity deficits.

Many of the studies summarized in this book were published in prestigious or high-impact journals such as the *Journal of the American Medical Association, New England Journal of Medicine, British Medical Journal, Annals of Medicine, Clinical Infectious Diseases, Emerging Infectious Diseases, Journal of Infectious Diseases, Journal of Internal Medicine, The Lancet, Pediatrics, Journal of Pediatrics, Pediatric Infectious Disease Journal, European Journal of Pediatrics, Vaccine, Epidemiology, American Journal of Epidemiology, European Journal of Epidemiology, International Journal of Cancer* and the *American Journal of Public Health.* Of course, this does not mean that studies published in highly-cited journals are more valuable than those published in lesser known journals. All studies must be scrutinized for potential strengths and weaknesses.

The scientific papers in this book are organized into 24 chapters. Each chapter contains several studies on a particular topic, such as aluminum adjuvants, pathogen evolution, sudden infant death, and healthcare workers who reject vaccines. Usually, there is one study per page although some pages contain two or three studies. At the top of each page is a headline. Next, there is a direct quote taken from the study. This is followed by the scientific citation. Finally, I use bullet points to summarize, in my own words, pertinent findings in the paper.

Many of the studies could have been included in other categories. For example, although there is a separate chapter on measles and MMR, there are numerous studies related to MMR in the chapters on allergies, seizures, thrombocytopenia, cancer, and vitamin A. If you are looking for information on a particular vaccine or subject that is not covered under a chapter heading, the index may be helpful.

Important findings from each scientific paper reviewed in this book are provided for quick reference and to counterbalance the many well-publicized studies touting the advantages of vaccination. I endeavored to remain free from bias at all times, with one caveat — my goal was to summarize studies that shed light on poorly publicized and unpopular aspects of vaccination. For readers with a scientific background, I included risk ratios, odds ratios, relative incidence and other statistical measures when p-values achieved significance. Confidence intervals can be found in the original studies.

Some of the summarized studies have favorable conclusions toward vaccines although actual findings in the paper are critical of vaccines. Authors of research papers often put a positive spin on studies with undesirable findings. Also, the findings in some of the summarized studies may conflict with those in other studies. There are many reasons why studies on the same topic might have contrary results. Studies may be poorly designed or conducted by researchers with conflicts of interest that bias their findings. This topic is discussed in the final chapter.

I highly recommend reading the actual complete studies, which often contain supplementary figures, tables, data and discussions not included in my summaries. Some scientific papers are freely available from the medical journals that published them. Others are fee-based although an abstract of the paper is almost always available at no cost.

Studies that support vaccination are not included in this book. You can find supportive information by visiting official websites of the Centers for Disease Control and Prevention (CDC), the Food and Drug Administration (FDA), the World Health Organization (WHO), vaccine manufacturers, and by conducting your own search in medical journals. I encourage you to do your own careful research to better understand the benefits and risks of vaccination.

Neil Z. Miller
Medical Research Journalist

Vaccination Schedules

The four studies in this chapter investigated safety issues associated with recommended vaccination schedules. The first study analyzed the vaccination schedules of 34 developed nations and found a significant correlation between infant mortality rates and the number of vaccine doses infants receive. Developed nations that require the most vaccines tend to have the worst infant mortality rates.

The second study analyzed 38,801 reports of infants who had adverse events after receiving vaccinations. Infants who received the most vaccines concurrently were significantly more likely to be hospitalized or die, when compared to infants who received fewer vaccines concurrently.

The third study compared fully vaccinated children to under-vaccinated children (they did not receive all vaccines as recommended). Children who were under-vaccinated the most had the fewest visits to a healthcare provider for upper respiratory illness and significantly lower rates of outpatient and emergency department visits, compared to on-time, fully vaccinated children.

In the fourth study, scientists administered age-adjusted pediatric vaccines to baby monkeys according to the complete U.S. recommended childhood vaccination schedule. The vaccinated primates had abnormalities in the region of the brain affecting social and emotional development, and a significant increase in total brain volume. An accelerated increase in total brain volume between 6 and 14 months of age is a consistent finding for many children with autism.

1.

Developed nations that require the most vaccines tend to have the worst infant mortality rates

"These findings demonstrate a counterintuitive relationship: nations that require more vaccine doses tend to have higher infant mortality rates. A closer inspection of correlations between vaccine doses, biochemical or synergistic toxicity, and infant mortality rates, is essential."

Miller NZ, Goldman GS. **Infant mortality rates regressed against number of vaccine doses routinely given: is there a biochemical or synergistic toxicity?** *Hum Exp Toxicol* 2011; 30(9): 1420-28.

- The U.S. requires infants to receive 26 vaccine doses, the most in the world, yet 33 nations have better infant mortality rates.

- This study analyzed the vaccination schedules of 34 developed nations and found a significant correlation between infant mortality rates and the number of vaccine doses infants receive. Nations that require the most vaccines tend to have the worst infant mortality rates.

- Linear regression analysis showed a high statistically significant link between increasing vaccine doses and increasing infant mortality rates ($r = 0.992$).

- Developed nations that require the least number of infant vaccines tend to have the best infant mortality rates.

- Many third world nations have high vaccination rates (above 90%) and require their infants to receive a high number of vaccine doses but their infant mortality rates are poor.

- Infant mortality rates remain high in developing nations that cannot furnish clean water, proper nutrition, good sanitation, and better access to health care.

- There is evidence that a subset of infants may be susceptible to sudden infant death shortly after receiving vaccines. Some vaccine-related infant deaths may be reclassified by medical authorities as ordinary mortality concealing a link between vaccines and fatalities.

2.

Infants who receive the most vaccines have the worst hospitalization and death rates

"Since vaccines are given to millions of infants annually, it is imperative that health authorities have scientific data from synergistic toxicity studies on all combinations of vaccines that infants might receive. Universal vaccine recommendations must be supported by such studies. Finding ways to increase vaccine safety should be the highest priority."

Goldman GS, Miller NZ. **Relative trends in hospitalizations and mortality among infants by the number of vaccine doses and age, based on the Vaccine Adverse Event Reporting System (VAERS), 1990-2010.** *Hum Exp Toxicol* 2012; 31(10): 1012-21.

- This study was designed to determine a) whether infants who receive several vaccines simultaneously rather than fewer are more likely to be hospitalized or die, and b) whether younger infants are more likely than older infants to be hospitalized or die after receiving vaccines.

- This study analyzed 38,801 reports of infants who had adverse events after receiving vaccinations. The reports were accessed from the FDA's Vaccine Adverse Event Reporting System (VAERS) database, 1990-2010.

- Infants who received 6, 7, or 8 vaccine doses were significantly more likely to be hospitalized when compared to infants who received 2, 3, or 4 vaccine doses ($r^2 = 0.91$). Younger infants were significantly more likely than older infants to be hospitalized after receiving vaccines ($r^2 = 0.95$).

- Infants who received 5-8 vaccine doses were significantly more likely to die when compared to infants who received 1-4 vaccine doses (rate ratio, RR= 1.5). Vaccinated infants under 6 months of age were significantly more likely to die than vaccinated infants aged 6 months to less than 1 year (RR = 3.0).

- Male infants were significantly more likely than female infants to die after receiving vaccines (RR = 1.4).

- The safety of combining multiple vaccines during a single physician visit as recommended by CDC guidelines was never affirmed in clinical studies.

3.

Fully vaccinated children are significantly more likely to require emergency care than under-vaccinated children

"Children who were under-vaccinated because of parental choice had significantly lower utilization rates of the emergency department and outpatient settings — both overall and for specific acute illnesses — than children who were vaccinated on time."

Glanz JM, Newcomer SR, et al. **A population-based cohort study of undervaccination in 8 managed care organizations across the United States.** *JAMA Pediatr* 2013 Mar 1; 167(3): 274-81.

- This study analyzed 323,247 healthcare records to compare children under 2 years of age who were fully vaccinated at CDC-recommended ages to children who were under-vaccinated (they did not receive all vaccines according to the recommended schedule).

- Children who were under-vaccinated the most had the greatest reductions in outpatient visits and healthcare utilization for upper respiratory illness, fever and pharyngitis when compared to on-time, fully vaccinated children (36% to 38% reductions).

- Children who were under-vaccinated because of parental choice had lower inpatient admission rates and significantly lower rates of outpatient and emergency department visits (incidence rate ratio, IRR = 0.94 and 0.91, respectively) compared to on-time, fully vaccinated children.

- Nearly half of the children in this study were under-vaccinated — a growing trend.

- About 13% of the children were under-vaccinated due to parental choice.

- All inpatient and emergency department visits between birth and 8 days of age were excluded from analysis although a hepatitis B vaccine is given to on-time, fully vaccinated children at birth.

4.

Baby monkeys that were given vaccines according to the U.S. vaccination schedule had abnormalities in the region of the brain affecting social and emotional development

"These results raise the possibility that multiple vaccine exposures during the previous 3-4 months may have had a significant impact on brain growth and development... [and] warrant additional research into the potential impact of an interaction between the MMR and thimerosal-containing vaccines on brain structure and function."

Hewitson L, Lopresti BJ, et al. **Influence of pediatric vaccines on amygdala growth and opioid ligand binding in rhesus macaque infants: a pilot study**. *Acta Neurobiol Exp* 2010; 70: 147-64.

- This study was designed to investigate structural and functional changes in the developing infant primate brain following administration of U.S. pediatric vaccines according to the recommended childhood schedule.
- In this study, 12 male infant rhesus macaques received the complete, age-adjusted childhood vaccine regimen. Four additional macaques, the control group, received saline injections. MRI and PET scans at 4 and 6 months of age were obtained from 9 of the vaccinated and 2 of the control animals.
- The MMR, DTaP, and Hib-vaccinated primates had significantly altered amygdala growth (associated with the development of social and emotional behavior) compared to the unvaccinated primates.
- The vaccinated primates had a significant increase in total brain volume. An accelerated increase in total brain volume between 6 and 14 months of age is a consistent finding for many children with autism.
- Findings in this study suggest that vaccines may be associated with significant disturbances in brain growth and development.

Thimerosal (Mercury)

Thimerosal contains mercury. It is added to multi-dose vials of vaccines to prevent bacterial contamination when more than one needle is inserted into the vial. In the United States, infants and children received high quantities of mercury from several CDC-recommended vaccines that contained thimerosal — DTaP, hepatitis B and *Haemophilus influenzae* type b (Hib) — until about 2002 when thimerosal was removed from most vaccines.

Today, developed countries continue to inject significant quantities of mercury from thimerosal-containing influenza vaccines into pregnant women, infants and children. In developing nations, infants are still exposed to high quantities of mercury from several thimerosal-containing vaccines. This dubious practice continues because the World Health Organization (WHO) estimated that it saves about 15 cents per vaccine dose to manufacture 10-dose vials (with thimerosal) compared to single-dose vials without mercury [*Bull World Health Organ* 2003; 81(10): 726-31].

The studies in this chapter provide strong evidence that vaccines containing mercury significantly increase the risk of neurodevelopmental effects, including speech and sleep disorders, developmental delay, attention deficit disorder, premature puberty, mental retardation, and autism.

5.

Infants who received vaccines containing mercury had significantly increased odds of being diagnosed with an autism spectrum disorder

"The present study provides new epidemiological evidence supporting an association between increasing organic-mercury exposure from thimerosal-containing childhood vaccines and the subsequent risk of an autism spectrum disorder diagnosis."

Geier DA, Hooker BS, et al. **A two-phase study evaluating the relationship between thimerosal-containing vaccine administration and the risk for an autism spectrum disorder diagnosis in the United States.** *Transl Neurodegener* 2013 Dec 19; 2(1): 25.

- Thimerosal contains mercury. It is added to some vaccines as a preservative.
- This study was designed to evaluate the toxic effects of mercury in childhood vaccines. Phase I analyzed the Vaccine Adverse Event Reporting System (VAERS) database (which is jointly maintained by the CDC and FDA) for reports of autism spectrum disorders following DTaP vaccination.
- Phase II of this study analyzed the Vaccine Safety Datalink (VSD) database (created by the CDC) to identify children with and without an autism spectrum disorder diagnosis — the cases and controls — and then compared their infant exposures to mercury from hepatitis B vaccines.
- The phase II study protocol was approved by the CDC.
- Infants who received DTaP vaccines with mercury had twice the risk for a subsequent autism spectrum disorder reported to VAERS compared to infants who received mercury-free DTaP vaccines (risk ratio, RR = 2.02).
- Infants who received 37.5 mcg of mercury from thimerosal-containing hepatitis B vaccines within the first six months of life were 3 times more likely to have subsequently been diagnosed with an autism spectrum disorder compared to those who received mercury-free hepatitis B vaccines (odds ratio, OR=3.39).

6.

Infants who received vaccines containing mercury developed speech disorders, sleep disorders and autism

"This analysis suggests that high exposure to ethylmercury from thimerosal-containing vaccines in the first month of life increases the risk of subsequent development of neurologic development impairment."

Verstraeten T, Davies R, et al. **Increased risk of developmental neurologic impairment after high exposure to thimerosal-containing vaccine in first month of life.** *Proceedings of the Epidemic Intelligence Service Annual Conference*, vol. 49 (Centers for Disease Control and Prevention; Atlanta, GA, USA, April 2000).

- This study was designed to determine whether infants who are exposed to ethylmercury from thimerosal-containing vaccines are at increased risk of degenerative and developmental neurologic disorders and renal disorders before the age of six.

- This study was conducted by the CDC using the Vaccine Safety Datalink (VSD) containing vaccination and demographic data on over 400,000 infants.

- The risk of developing a neurologic development disorder was nearly twice as high (RR = 1.8) in infants who received the highest cumulative exposure to ethylmercury (> 25 mcg) from thimerosal-containing vaccines at 1 month of age when compared to infants who were unexposed to mercury.

- One-month-old infants with the highest cumulative exposure to ethylmercury also had twice the risk of developing a speech disorder, 5 times the risk of developing a non-organic sleep disorder, and were 7.6 times more likely to develop autism when compared to infants who were unexposed to mercury from thimerosal-containing vaccines.

- Premature babies were excluded from this study.

- There was no increased risk for neurologic degenerative and renal disorders.

- This study was never published.

7.

Neurodevelopmental disorders are significantly more common in children who received vaccines containing mercury

"This study provides new epidemiological evidence supporting a significant relationship between increasing organic-mercury exposure from thimerosal-containing vaccines and the subsequent risk of a neurodevelopmental disorder diagnosis."

Geier DA, Hooker BS, et al. **A dose-response relationship between organic mercury exposure from thimerosal-containing vaccines and neurodevelopmental disorders.** *Int J Environ Res Public Health* 2014 Sep 5; 11(9): 9156-70.

- This study examined the medical records of more than 1.9 million infants enrolled in the CDC's Vaccine Safety Datalink (VSD) project to determine whether exposure to mercury from thimerosal-containing vaccines influences the risk of neurodevelopmental disorders.

- Children who were diagnosed with neurodevelopmental disorders were matched to a control group. Each child was then assessed for cumulative mercury exposure from thimerosal-containing hepatitis B vaccines administered within the first 6 months of life.

- Children who were exposed to the most mercury (37.5 mcg) were significantly more likely than controls to have been diagnosed with pervasive developmental disorder (OR = 3.0), specific developmental delay (OR = 2.3), tic disorder (OR = 2.2) or hyperkinetic syndrome of childhood (OR = 2.9).

- It is imperative that health authorities end the practice of adding thimerosal to vaccines.

- The study protocol was approved by the CDC.

8.

Developmental delays are 3 times more common in children who received vaccines with mercury

"The present study provides compelling new epidemiological evidence supporting a significant relationship between increasing organic-mercury exposure from thimerosal-containing childhood vaccines and the subsequent risk of a diagnosis for specific delays in development among both males and females."

Geier DA, Kern JK, et al. **Thimerosal-containing hepatitis b vaccination and the risk for diagnosed specific delays in development in the United States: A case-control study in the vaccine safety datalink.** *North Am J Med Sci* 2014; 6: 519-31.

- This study compared 5,699 children diagnosed with developmental delays to 48,528 children without delays in development to determine the cumulative amount of mercury they received from vaccines within their first, second, and sixth months of life.

- Children who were diagnosed with speech/language, coordination, hearing, and reading disorders were significantly more likely to have received 12.5, 25, and 37.5 mcg of mercury from thimerosal-containing vaccines within the first, second, and sixth months of life (odds ratios, OR = 1.99, 1.98, 3.07), respectively, compared to 0 mcg of mercury in the control group.

- Children who received three thimerosal-containing hepatitis B vaccines within the first six months of life — as recommended by the CDC — were diagnosed with developmental delays at a rate 3 times greater than children who did not receive thimerosal-containing hepatitis B vaccines.

- Exposure to mercury from thimerosal-containing vaccines during early infancy is a significant risk factor among males and females for a later diagnosis of developmental delays.

- The study protocol was approved by the CDC.

9.

Psychomotor development — the ability to crawl, walk, and run — is adversely affected by neonatal exposure to thimerosal-containing vaccines

"Our results have shown that ethylmercury is not completely harmless for the first stage of life and may be responsible for poorer outcomes of psychomotor development in children."

Mrozek-Budzyn D, Majewska R, et al. **Neonatal exposure to thimerosal from vaccines and child development in the first 3 years of life.** *Neurotoxicol Teratol* 2012 Nov-Dec; 34(6): 592-97.

- This study was designed to determine whether child development is affected by early infant exposure to thimerosal-containing vaccines.
- Newborns who received thimerosal-containing hepatitis B vaccines were compared to newborns who received thimerosal-free hepatitis B vaccines. Additional exposures to thimerosal-containing vaccines up to 6 months of age were also examined.
- At 12 months and 24 months of age, psychomotor development (muscle control over the ability to crawl, sit, stand, walk, run, and jump) in neonates who received thimerosal-containing vaccines was significantly worse when compared to neonates unexposed to thimerosal-containing vaccines.
- Over the course of the 3-year follow-up, overall psychomotor deficits were significantly worse in neonates exposed to thimerosal-containing vaccines.
- The authors of this study believe that adverse consequences, such as delays in psychomotor development, could be avoided by removing thimerosal from vaccines.

10.

Boys who received hepatitis B vaccines with mercury were 9 times more likely than unvaccinated boys to become developmentally disabled

"This study found statistically significant evidence to suggest that boys in the United States who were vaccinated with the triple series hepatitis B vaccine, during the time period in which vaccines were manufactured with thimerosal, were more susceptible to developmental disability than were unvaccinated boys."

Gallagher C, Goodman M. **Hepatitis B triple series vaccine and developmental disability in US children aged 1-9 years.** *Toxicol Environ Chem* 2008 Sep-Oct; 90(5): 997-1008.

- In 1991, the CDC recommended that all U.S. infants receive 3 doses of a new hepatitis B vaccine made with mercury, with the first dose beginning at birth. From 1991 to 1999, the number of children requiring special education services for autism increased by 500%.
- This study investigated the link between developmental disability in children 1-9 years of age and prior infant vaccination with 3 doses of the newly recommended mercury-containing hepatitis B vaccine.
- Boys who received 3 doses of the mercury-containing hepatitis B vaccine during infancy were nearly 9 times more likely (OR = 8.63) than unvaccinated boys to need early intervention services, a proxy for developmental disability.
- This study provides strong evidence toward answering the Institute of Medicine's open question about whether there is a link between mercury-containing vaccines and neurodevelopmental disorders.
- In developing nations, hepatitis B (and other) vaccines still contain mercury. In the United States, some influenza vaccines still contain mercury.

11.

Boys who received hepatitis B vaccines containing mercury were 3 times more likely than unvaccinated boys to develop autism

"Boys vaccinated as neonates had threefold greater odds for autism diagnosis compared to boys never vaccinated or vaccinated after the first month of life."

Gallagher CM, Goodman MS. **Hepatitis B vaccination of male neonates and autism diagnosis, NHIS 1997-2002.** *J Toxicol Environ Health A* 2010; 73(24): 1665-77.

- Prior to 1999, hepatitis B vaccines administered at birth contained mercury.
- This study compared infants who received a mercury-containing hepatitis B vaccine within the first 4 weeks of life to infants who never received a hepatitis B vaccine or received it when they were older.
- Boys aged 3 to 17 years, who were born prior to 1999 and received a mercury-containing hepatitis B vaccine in their first month of life, were 3 times more likely to have been diagnosed with autism compared to boys who were never vaccinated or vaccinated later (odds ratio, OR = 3.0).
- Infants in this study were vaccinated before thimerosal-free vaccines became available, so possible adverse effects associated with thimerosal in the hepatitis B vaccines they received is a serious concern.
- More than 5 boys were diagnosed with autism for every autistic girl.
- Non-white boys had the greatest risk of autism.
- Children without a vaccination record were excluded from this study, so the prevalence of an autism diagnosis may be underestimated.

12.

Autism, mental retardation, and speech disorders were significantly more common in children who received DTaP vaccines with thimerosal

"The present study provides additional compelling epidemiological evidence supporting a significant relationship between increased organic-mercury exposure from Thimerosal-preserved childhood vaccines and the subsequent risk of a neurodevelopmental diagnosis."

Geier DA, Kern JK, et al. **The risk of neurodevelopmental disorders following a Thimerosal-preserved DTaP formulation in comparison to its Thimerosal-reduced formulation in the Vaccine Adverse Event Reporting System (VAERS).** *J Biochem Pharmacol Res* 2014 Jun; 2(2): 64-73.

- This study analyzed 5,591 adverse event reports in the VAERS database to determine whether reports of neurodevelopmental disorders were more likely in children who received DTaP vaccines with thimerosal (administered from 1997-1999) or without thimerosal (administered from 2004-2006).

- Children who received DTaP vaccines with thimerosal were significantly more likely to develop autism (odds ratio, OR = 7.67), mental retardation (OR = 8.73), speech disorders (OR = 3.49), or neurodevelopmental disorders (OR = 4.82) than children who received thimerosal-reduced DTaP vaccines.

- During the 1990s, infants in the U.S. received up to 200 mcg of mercury from thimerosal-containing vaccines during the first 6 months of life.

- In the U.S., babies in utero, infants, children and pregnant women still receive substantial amounts of mercury from thimerosal-containing influenza vaccines. In many developing nations, thimerosal-preserved childhood vaccines still remain a substantial source of mercury exposure for infants.

- The findings in this study are supported by several previous epidemiological studies. It is a public health imperative to "do no harm" by removing mercury from all vaccines.

13.

Autism, mental retardation and personality disorders occurred more often in children who received vaccines with thimerosal

"This study provides additional epidemiological evidence for a link between increasing mercury from thimerosal-containing childhood vaccines and neurodevelopmental disorders."

Geier DA, Geier MR. **An assessment of the impact of thimerosal on childhood neurodevelopmental disorders.** *Pediatr Rehabil* 2003 Apr-Jun; 6(2): 97-102.

- This study analyzed the Vaccine Adverse Event Reporting System (VAERS) database, data from the U.S. Department of Education, and FDA safety guidelines for the oral ingestion of methylmercury, to assess whether mercury in childhood vaccines contributed to neurodevelopmental disorders.

- Analyzing VAERS, children who received DTaP vaccines with thimerosal were significantly more likely to develop autism (OR = 2.6), mental retardation (OR = 2.5), and personality disorders (OR = 1.5) when compared to children who received thimerosal-free DTaP vaccines.

- For every additional microgram (mcg) of mercury injected into a child via thimerosal-containing vaccines, the odds of developing autism increased by 2.9%, mental retardation increased by 4.8%, and personality disorders increased by 1.2%.

- Data from the U.S. Department of Education revealed a significant relationship between increasing mercury from thimerosal in childhood vaccines and autism (OR = 2.5) and speech disorders (OR = 1.4).

- Compared to FDA safety guidelines for the daily oral ingestion of methylmercury, children received up to 32 times more mercury than allowable from their childhood vaccines.

- The findings in this study and others indicate that thimerosal should be removed immediately from all childhood vaccines.

14.

Rates of autism and mental retardation were 6 times higher in children who received DTaP vaccines with thimerosal

"This study presents the first epidemiologic evidence, based upon tens of millions of doses of vaccine administered in the United States, that associates increasing thimerosal from vaccines with neuro-developmental disorders."

Geier MR, Geier DA. **Neurodevelopmental disorders after thimerosal-containing vaccines: a brief communication.** *Exp Biol Med (Maywood)* 2003 Jun; 228(6): 660-64.

- The U.S. Vaccine Adverse Events Reporting System (VAERS) database was analyzed for possible correlations between receipt of thimerosal-containing vaccines and neurodevelopmental disorders.
- The incidence rate of autism and mental retardation was 6 times higher, and speech disorders were twice as likely to occur, in children who received DTaP vaccines with thimerosal compared to thimerosal-free DTaP vaccines.

15.

Geier D, Geier MR. **Neurodevelopmental disorders following thimerosal-containing childhood immunizations: a follow-up analysis.** *Int J Toxicol* 2004 Nov-Dec; 23(6): 369-76.

"The present study provides additional epidemiological evidence supporting previous epidemiological, clinical and experimental evidence that administration of thimerosal-containing vaccines in the United States resulted in a significant number of children developing neuro-developmental disorders."

- Children who received DTaP vaccines containing thimerosal were significantly more likely than children who received thimerosal-free DTaP vaccines to have adverse events reported to VAERS for autism, mental retardation, speech disorder, personality disorder, and thinking abnormality.

16.

Risks of autism, mental retardation and personality disorders significantly increased in children who received vaccines containing thimerosal

"Significantly increased adjusted risks of autism, speech disorders, mental retardation, personality disorders, thinking abnormalities, ataxia, and neurodevelopmental disorders in general, with minimal systematic error or confounding, were associated with thimerosal-containing vaccine exposure."

Geier DA, Geier MR. **A meta-analysis epidemiological assessment of neurodevelopmental disorders following vaccines administered from 1994 through 2000 in the United States.** *Neuro Endocrinol Lett* 2006 Aug; 27(4): 401-13.

- This paper found significant links between thimerosal-containing vaccines, which contain ethylmercury, and reported neurodevelopmental disorders.

17.

Geier DA, Geier MR. **A comparative evaluation of the effects of MMR immunization and mercury doses from thimerosal-containing childhood vaccines on the population prevalence of autism.** *Med Sci Monit* 2004 Mar; 10(3): PI33-9.

"There is biological plausibility and epidemiological evidence showing a direct relationship between increasing doses of mercury from thimerosal-containing vaccines and neurodevelopmental disorders, and measles-containing vaccines and serious neurological disorders. It is recommended that thimerosal be removed from all vaccines, and additional research be undertaken to produce an MMR vaccine with an improved safety profile."

- Children who received increasing doses of mercury from thimerosal-containing vaccines were significantly more likely to develop autism when compared to a baseline measurement.

18.

There is a significant relationship between regressive autism spectrum disorders and the amount of mercury children received from thimerosal-containing vaccines

"It is clear that while genetic factors are important to the pathogenesis of autism spectrum disorders (ASDs), mercury exposure can induce immune, sensory, neurological, motor, and behavioral dysfunctions similar to traits defining or associated with ASDs."

Geier DA, Geier MR. **A case series of children with apparent mercury toxic encephalopathies manifesting with clinical symptoms of regressive autistic disorders.** *J Toxicol Environ Health A* 2007 May 15; 70(10): 837-51.

- This paper describes genetic and developmental evaluations of nine children with regressive autism spectrum disorders.

- Eight of the nine children excreted large amounts of mercury after chelation therapy, had no known exposure to mercury except from thimerosal-containing vaccines and/or Rho(D)-immune globulin given during fetal growth, and had other possible causes for their regressive autism ruled out.

- There was a significant relationship between the total amount of mercury the children received and the severity of their regressive autism.

- Following their exposure to significant quantities of mercury from thimerosal-containing vaccines and/or Rho(D)-immune globulin during their fetal/infant growth, these children suffered from mercury toxic encephalopathies between the ages of 1 and 2 years that manifested with symptoms of regressive autism.

- The study protocol was approved by the U.S. Department of Health and Human Services.

19.

A CDC-sponsored database shows significant links between thimerosal in vaccines and neurodevelopmental disabilities, including autism and ADD

"This study showed that exposure to mercury from thimerosal-containing vaccines administered in the U.S. was a consistent significant risk factor for the development of neurodevelopmental disorders."

Geier DA, Geier MR. **A two-phased population epidemiological study of the safety of thimerosal-containing vaccines: a follow-up analysis.** *Med Sci Monit* 2005 Apr; 11(4): CR160-70.

- This study analyzed a) VAERS for possible neurodevelopmental effects of thimerosal-containing DTaP vaccines, and b) the Vaccine Safety Datalink (VSD) for the risk of neurodevelopmental disorders from cumulative exposures to mercury from thimerosal-containing vaccines.

- Receipt of thimerosal-containing vaccines was associated with significantly increased risks for autism, mental retardation, developmental delays, language delays, attention deficit disorder (ADD), and tics.

20.

Young HA, Geier DA, et al. **Thimerosal exposure in infants and neuro-developmental disorders: an assessment of computerized medical records in the Vaccine Safety Datalink.** *J Neurol Sci* 2008 Aug 15; 271(1-2): 110-18.

"Consistent significantly increased rate ratios were observed for autism, autism spectrum disorders, tics, attention deficit disorder, and emotional disturbances with mercury exposure from thimerosal-containing vaccines."

- This study examined the medical records of 278,624 children in the CDC-sponsored Vaccine Safety Datalink (VSD) and found significant associations between mercury-containing vaccines and neurodevelopmental disorders.

21.

Young mice and rats injected with thimerosal (mercury) had behavioral impairments characteristic of autistic children

"Neonatal exposure to a higher dose of thimerosal-mercury caused autistic- and depressive-like behaviors in adult mice, suggesting long-lasting adverse effects in mouse brains."

Li X, Qu F, et al. **Transcriptomic analyses of neurotoxic effects in mouse brain after intermittent neonatal administration of thimerosal.** *Toxicol Sci* 2014 Jun; 139(2): 452-65.

- Thimerosal-injected mice showed substantial neurodevelopmental delay, social interaction deficiency, synaptic dysfunction, and impairment of the endocrine system, manifesting as autistic-like behavior.
- The prefrontal cortex and temporal cortex of thimerosal-injected mouse brains had "dark" neurons that were dying.

22.

Olczak M, Duszczyk M, et al. **Persistent behavioral impairments and alterations of brain dopamine system after early postnatal administration of thimerosal in rats.** *Behav Brain Res* 2011 Sep 30; 223(1): 107-18.

"These data document that early postnatal thimerosal administration causes lasting neurobehavioral impairments and neurochemical alterations in the brain, dependent on dose and sex. If similar changes occur in thimerosal/mercurial-exposed children, they could contribute to neurodevelopmental disorders."

- This study injected young rats with thimerosal to investigate its effects on behaviors which are typically found in autistic children.
- Thimerosal-injected rats had impaired locomotion, increased anxiety and more antisocial interactions.

23.

Young rats injected with thimerosal in doses equivalent to those used in infant vaccines developed severe brain pathologies

"These findings document neurotoxic effects of thimerosal, at doses equivalent to those used in infant vaccines or higher, in developing rat brain, suggesting likely involvement of this mercurial in neurodevelopmental disorders."

Olczak M, Duszczyk M, et al. **Lasting neuropathological changes in rat brain after intermittent neonatal administration of thimerosal.** *Folia Neuropathol* 2010; 48(4): 258-69.

- Thimerosal, which contains mercury and is added to some childhood vaccines, is suspected of causing iatrogenic complications that might contribute to childhood neurodevelopmental disorders including autism.
- This study injected baby rats with thimerosal in doses similar to those used in human infant vaccines to study its effects on brain pathology.
- Several neuropathologies were observed, including neuron degeneration, reduced synaptic reactions, and atrophy in the hippocampus and cerebellum.

24.

Olczak M, Duszczyk M, et al. **Neonatal administration of thimerosal causes persistent changes in mu opioid receptors in the rat brain.** *Neurochem Res* 2010 Nov; 35(11): 1840-7.

"These data document that exposure to thimerosal during early postnatal life produces lasting alterations in the densities of brain opioid receptors along with other neuropathological changes, which may disturb brain development."

- Young rats were injected with thimerosal and their brains examined. Neuropathologies included neuron degeneration and loss of synaptic integrity.

25.

Brain injuries can be induced in rats by injecting them with thimerosal

"The current study provides further empirical evidence that exposure to thimerosal leads to neurotoxic changes in the developing brain, arguing for urgent and permanent removal of this preservative from all vaccines for children (and adults) since effective, less toxic and less costly alternatives are available. The stubborn insistence of some vaccine manufacturers and health agencies on continuation of use of this proven neurotoxin in vaccines is testimony of their disregard for both the health of young generations and for the environment."

Duszczyk-Budhathoki M, Olczak M, et al. **Administration of thimerosal to infant rats increases overflow of glutamate and aspartate in the prefrontal cortex: protective role of dehydroepiandrosterone sulfate.** *Neurochem Res* 2012 Feb; 37(2): 436-47.

- This study injected rats with thimerosal to examine the effect on extracellular levels of neuroactive amino acids in the prefrontal cortex.
- Rats injected with thimerosal had increased glutamate and aspartate in the prefrontal cortex suggesting that neonatal exposure to thimerosal-containing vaccines could induce brain injuries and neurodevelopmental disorders.

26.

Sulkowski ZL, Chen T, et al. **Maternal thimerosal exposure results in aberrant cerebellar oxidative stress, thyroid hormone metabolism, and motor behavior in rat pups; sex- and strain-dependent effects.** *Cerebellum* 2012 Jun; 11(2): 575-86.

"Our data demonstrate a negative neurodevelopmental impact of perinatal thimerosal exposure."

- In this study, pregnant and lactating rats were injected with thimerosal to evaluate its effect on their neonates. Thimerosal exposure in rat moms caused a delayed startle response and decreased motor learning in their babies. It also significantly increased cerebellar levels of oxidative stress.

27.

Newborn monkeys that received a thimerosal-containing hepatitis B vaccine had significant delays in neonatal reflexes and neurological development

"This primate model provides a possible means of assessing adverse neurodevelopmental outcomes from neonatal thimerosal-containing hepatitis B vaccine exposure, particularly in infants of lower gestational age or birth weight."

Hewitson L, Houser LA, et al. **Delayed acquisition of neonatal reflexes in newborn primates receiving a thimerosal-containing hepatitis B vaccine: influence of gestational age and birth weight.** *J Toxicol Environ Health A.* 2010; 73(19): 1298-1313.

- The purpose of this study was to determine whether acquisition of reflexes in newborn rhesus macaques is affected by receipt of a neonatal dose of a thimerosal-containing hepatitis B vaccine.

- A weight-adjusted thimerosal-containing hepatitis B vaccine was given to male macaques within 24 hours of birth. A control group of unexposed macaques received either a saline placebo or no injection.

- The newborn primates were tested daily for acquisition of nine survival, motor, and sensorimotor reflexes. Exposed primates had a significant delay in the acquisition of root, snout, and suck reflexes, compared with unexposed primates. No reflexes were significantly delayed in unexposed primates.

- Lower birth weight and/or lower gestational age increased the adverse effects following vaccine exposure.

- Although primate testing is an important component of pre-clinical safety assessment of vaccines intended for human use, the results found in this study are not included in current CDC recommendations for hepatitis B vaccine safety testing.

28.

Infants with the least exposure to fish methylmercury but the most exposure to vaccine ethylmercury had the worst neurodevelopmental behavior

"In nurslings whose mothers are exposed to different levels of fish methylmercury...neurological development at six months was negatively associated with exposure to additional ethylmercury [from] thimerosal-containing vaccines."

Dórea JG, Marques RC, Isejima C. **Neurodevelopment of Amazonian infants: antenatal and postnatal exposure to methyl- and ethylmercury.** *J Biomed Biotechnol* 2012; 2012:132876.

- Amazonian babies are exposed to methylmercury (abundant in maternal fish diets during pregnancy and breastfeeding) and ethylmercury from thimerosal-containing vaccines.

- Scientists visited three different Amazonian communities (one urban center and two rural villages) to compare neurobehavioral development — motor skills, language development, adaptive behavior and personal social behavior — in 6-month-old infants who were exposed to varying combinations of fish methylmercury and vaccine-related ethylmercury.

- Infants from the Amazonian community with the lowest exposure to fish methylmercury but the highest exposure to vaccine-related ethylmercury had the worst cumulative neurodevelopmental scores.

- This study revealed a significant association between infants who are exposed to environmental fish methylmercury and iatrogenic vaccine ethylmercury and neurobehavioral deficits.

- The thimerosal-containing vaccines — hepatitis B and DTP — given to the infants also contained aluminum salts as an adjuvant, so the ethylmercury and aluminum salts were treated as a unit.

29.

There is abundant evidence that thimerosal-containing vaccines are neurotoxic and should not be given to pregnant women or children

"Thimerosal-containing vaccines continue to be administered on a regular basis to potentially the most vulnerable populations: pregnant women and children (especially in developing countries). Given this, we believe it is high time to reassess the rationale for using thimerosal, a known immune and neurotoxic substance, in human vaccines."

Tomljenovic L, Dórea JG, et al. **Commentary: a link between mercury exposure, autism spectrum disorder, and other neurodevelopmental disorders? Implications for thimerosal-containing vaccines.** *Journal on Developmental Disabilities* 2012; 18(1): 34-42.

- Studies show a significant association between thimerosal-containing vaccines given to children and neurodevelopmental disorders, including autism, mental retardation, speech disorders and personality disorders.

- The U.S. Environmental Protection Agency limits mercury in drinking water to 2 parts per billion (ppb). Liquids with 200 ppb are classified as hazardous waste. Vaccines with "trace" amounts of thimerosal contain 600 ppb. Vaccines with full amounts of thimerosal contain mercury at 25,000 to 50,000 ppb.

- Mercury from thimerosal-containing vaccines accumulates in the brain.

- In the U.S. and Canada, pregnant women and children receive annual influenza vaccines, most of which contain full amounts of thimerosal. In Canada, many newborns receive hepatitis B vaccines with full amounts of thimerosal.

- Vaccine safety studies deliberately exclude vulnerable populations with pre-existing conditions but these people are encouraged to receive vaccines.

- There is abundant evidence that mercury from thimerosal in vaccines can be dangerous, especially to fetuses, infants and children. Its use in vaccines should be reconsidered.

30.

Children with autism were significantly more likely than controls to have mothers who received thimerosal-containing Rho(D) immune globulin during pregnancy

"The results provide insights into the potential role prenatal mercury exposure may play in some children with autism spectrum disorders."

Geier DA, Geier MR. **A prospective study of thimerosal-containing Rho(D)-immune globulin administration as a risk factor for autistic disorders.** *J Matern Fetal Neonatal Med* 2007 May; 20(5): 385-90.

- Starting in the late 1980s/early 1990s, Rho(D)-immune globulin was routinely given to all Rh-negative pregnant women at 28 weeks of gestation. Prior to 2002, most formulations of Rho(D) immune globulin contained thimerosal.
- This study investigated whether children with autism were more likely than controls to have been exposed to mercury in utero from thimerosal-containing Rho(D) immune globulin that RH-negative mothers receive during pregnancy.
- Children with autism spectrum disorders were significantly more likely than controls to have Rh-negative mothers (odds ratio, OR = 2.35). Researchers confirmed that each mother of a child with autism had received a thimerosal-containing Rho(D) immune globulin during her pregnancy.

31.

Geier DA, Mumper E, et al. **Neurodevelopmental disorders, maternal Rh-negativity, and Rho(D) immune globulins: a multi-center assessment.** *Neuro Endocrinol Lett* 2008 Apr; 29(2): 272-80.

"There were significant and comparable increases in maternal Rh-negativity among children with neurodevelopmental disorders, autism spectrum disorders, and attention-deficit-disorder/attention-deficit-hyperactivity-disorder...in comparison to both control groups. This study associates thimerosal-containing Rho(D) immune globulin with some neurodevelopmental disorders in children."

32.

180 studies provide evidence that thimerosal is dangerous; thimerosal-containing vaccines are unsafe for humans

"The culmination of the research that examines the effects of Thimerosal in humans indicates that it is a poison at minute levels with a plethora of deleterious consequences, even at the levels currently administered in vaccines."

Geier DA, King PG, et al. **Thimerosal: clinical, epidemiologic and biochemical studies.** *Clin Chim Acta* 2015 Apr 15; 444: 212-20.

- Thimerosal is a mercury-containing preservative that is still being used in some cosmetics, drugs and vaccines.

- At least 180 studies show that thimerosal is harmful. This paper reviewed clinical, epidemiological, and biochemical studies demonstrating adverse effects from human exposure to thimerosal and its ethylmercury components.

- Although reduced-thimerosal vaccines replaced thimerosal-preserved vaccines from 1999 through the early 2000s, in 2002 the CDC recommended influenza vaccines (with thimerosal) for infants, children and pregnant women.

- Most influenza vaccines still contain thimerosal. Compared to the CDC's pre-2000 recommended vaccination schedule, the maximum lifetime exposure to thimerosal from vaccines has actually increased.

- In developing nations, thimerosal is still used in many childhood vaccines and pregnant women are given thimerosal-containing tetanus vaccines.

- Studies show that thimerosal-containing vaccines given to pregnant women significantly increase thc risk of birth defects and fetal death.

- Several studies provide evidence that infant exposure to thimerosal-containing vaccines increases the risk of neurodevelopmental disorders, including autism spectrum disorder, attention deficit disorder and tic disorder. Other studies show that thimerosal is toxic to human neuron cells in vitro.

33.

Mercury in childhood vaccines can cause premature puberty

"The results of the present study show an association between increased mercury exposure from thimerosal-containing vaccines and premature puberty. The observed effects were consistent with the known human endocrine disrupting effects of mercury exposure."

Geier DA, Young HA, et al. **Thimerosal exposure and increasing trends of premature puberty in the vaccine safety datalink.** *Indian J Med Res* 2010 Apr; 131: 500-507.

- Mercury is a known endocrine disruptor that may interact with sex steroids to increase the risk of a child developing premature puberty. Many children with this condition, especially boys, are more aggressive than normal, which can cause behavior problems.

- This study used the CDC's Vaccine Safety Datalink (VSD) to evaluate the medical records of 278,624 children to determine if there is a relationship between varying levels of mercury from thimerosal-containing vaccines and the risk of developing premature puberty.

- This study found a statistically significant link between the amount of mercury infants received from thimerosal-containing vaccines and premature puberty.

- Infants who received an additional 100 mcg of mercury from their vaccines during the first seven months of life had a 5-fold increase (rate ratio, RR=5.58) in their risk of developing premature puberty.

- In this study, the median age of children diagnosed with premature puberty was 4.5 years, which is significantly younger than normal.

- This study found that 1 in 250 children has premature puberty, a 40-fold increase over previous estimates by the National Institutes of Health.

- Thimerosal should be removed from all vaccines as soon as possible.

- The study protocol was approved by the CDC.

34.

Six CDC studies showing that mercury in vaccines is safe are unreliable and provide evidence of scientific malfeasance

"The authors' decision to withhold data resembles scientific malfeasance."

Hooker B, Kern J, et al. **Methodological issues and evidence of malfeasance in research purporting to show thimerosal in vaccines is safe.** *BioMed Research International* 2014; article ID 247218.

- More than 165 studies examined thimerosal (a mercury-based compound added to many childhood vaccines) and found it to be harmful, yet the CDC insists that thimerosal is safe and there is no link between thimerosal-containing vaccines and autism.

- The CDC's claim that thimerosal is safe and that it does not cause autism is based on six studies that were coauthored and sponsored by the CDC.

- The purpose of this paper was to analyze these six CDC-sponsored studies and determine why their conclusions contradict the results of other investigations by numerous independent scientists over the past 75 years who have consistently found thimerosal to be harmful.

- The 6 studies analyzed in this paper, which were funded and overseen by the CDC — especially the studies showing a *protective* effect of thimerosal — have several methodological problems. For example, three of the studies withheld important results from the final publication.

- In a 7th study conducted directly by the CDC, infants who received thimerosal-containing vaccines were 7.6 times more likely to develop autism when compared to infants who were not exposed to thimerosal. The CDC failed to publicize or acknowledge this paper and its highly significant findings.

- The CDC has a conflict of interest (or research bias) because it sponsors vaccine studies while vaccine promotion is a central mission.

Aluminum

Aluminum is an adjuvant added into many vaccines to help stimulate a stronger immune response and increase vaccine efficacy. In the United States, Canada, the United Kingdom, Australia and many other nations, infants and children receive high quantities of aluminum from multiple injections of several vaccines. For example, vaccines for tetanus, pertussis (DTaP), *Haemophilus influenzae* type b (Hib), hepatitis A, hepatitis B, and pneumococcus contain aluminum.

Aluminum is neurotoxic, capable of destroying neurons necessary for proper cognitive and motor functions. After it is injected into the body it can travel to other organs and remain there for several years. The immune-stimulating effect of aluminum adjuvants can provoke autoimmune and inflammatory adverse reactions. Autoimmune disease and neurological damage can be induced in animals by injecting them with aluminum adjuvants.

The studies in this chapter provide strong evidence that aluminum adjuvants in vaccines significantly increase the risk of autoimmune disease and neurological disorders, including macrophagic myofasciitis, chronic fatigue, muscle weakness, cognitive deficits such as memory loss, sleep disturbances, and multiple sclerosis-like demyelinating central nervous system disorders. The immune-stimulating properties of aluminum adjuvants in vaccines also have similarities with several autoimmune/inflammatory diseases such as arthritis, type 1 diabetes, inflammatory bowel disease, lupus, and autism spectrum disorders.

35.

Aluminum in vaccines can cause autoimmune and neurological damage

"Hyperstimulation of the immune system by various [vaccine] adjuvants, including aluminum, carries an inherent risk for serious autoimmune disorders affecting the central nervous system."

Shaw CA, Tomljenovic L. **Aluminum in the central nervous system (CNS): toxicity in humans and animals, vaccine adjuvants, and autoimmunity.** *Immunol Res* 2013 Jul; 56(2-3): 304-16.

- This paper examined the evidence on aluminum neurotoxicity, particularly when added to vaccines as an adjuvant and injected into humans to stimulate an immune response.

- The immune-stimulating effect of aluminum adjuvants can provoke autoimmune and inflammatory adverse reactions.

- The medical and scientific literature provides ample evidence that aluminum is harmful to the nervous system in children and adults.

- Animal studies confirm that aluminum adjuvants can cause symptoms similar to amyotrophic lateral sclerosis (ALS), a progressive neurodegenerative disease that attacks nerve cells in the brain and spinal cord.

- There is a significant correlation between the number of aluminum-containing vaccines that children receive and the rate of autism spectrum disorders.

- Western countries that require the most aluminum-adjuvanted vaccines for preschool children have the highest autism rates.

- Injected aluminum is worse than ingested aluminum (from dietary sources) because it bypasses the protective barriers of the gastrointestinal tract, requiring a lower dose to induce a toxic reaction.

- The FDA never tested the safety of aluminum in childhood vaccines.

36.

Aluminum in vaccines may cause severe health problems in children and adults

"The continued use of aluminum adjuvants in various vaccines for children as well as the general public may be of significant concern. In particular, aluminum presented in this form carries a risk for autoimmunity, long-term brain inflammation and associated neurological complications and may thus have profound and widespread adverse health consequences."

Tomljenovic L, Shaw CA. **Aluminum vaccine adjuvants: are they safe?** *Curr Med Chem* 2011; 18(17): 2630-37.

- This paper summarizes what is currently known about aluminum toxicity and aluminum vaccine adjuvants.
- Aluminum is a neurotoxin and may be a co-factor in several neurodegenerative disorders and diseases, including Alzheimer's, Parkinson's, amyotrophic lateral sclerosis (ALS), multiple sclerosis, autism, and epilepsy.
- Aluminum adjuvants have the potential to induce serious immunological and neurological disorders in humans.
- Infants in the United States and other developed nations receive up to 49 times more aluminum from vaccines than FDA safety limits allow.
- Repeated injections of aluminum-containing vaccines in children may cause severe long-term immune system damage.
- No studies have been conducted to confirm the safety of combining aluminum with other toxic substances in vaccines, such as mercury, formaldehyde, phenoxyethanol, polysorbate 80, and glutaraldehyde.
- The FDA allows scientists conducting clinical trials to compare the safety of an aluminum-containing vaccine to an aluminum-containing "placebo." This underestimates the true rate of adverse vaccine reactions.
- Vaccine risks may exceed the potential benefits.

37.

Aluminum in vaccines may be linked to autism spectrum disorders

"Our results...suggest that a causal relationship may exist between the amount of aluminum administered to preschool children at various ages through vaccination and the rising prevalence of autism spectrum disorders."

Tomljenovic L, Shaw CA. **Do aluminum vaccine adjuvants contribute to the rising prevalence of autism?** *J Inorg Biochem* 2011 Nov; 105(11): 1489-99.

- Aluminum is extremely neurotoxic, capable of inducing neurological and immunological disorders in both animals and humans.

- Children in developed nations are exposed to significant amounts of aluminum adjuvants through vaccination programs. Such high exposures are repeated over short intervals during critical periods of brain development.

- This paper investigated whether aluminum added to childhood vaccines is contributing to the rising prevalence of autism spectrum disorders.

- There is a statistically significant correlation between the amount of aluminum infants receive from their vaccines and the rates of autism spectrum disorders in several developed nations (Pearson r = 0.89–0.94).

- Nations with the highest prevalence of autism spectrum disorders (U.S., U.K., Canada and Australia) require their children to receive the highest quantities of aluminum from vaccines, especially between 2 and 4 months of age.

- Repeated injections of aluminum in rats damaged their brains. Children in the U.S. are exposed to comparable quantities of aluminum from vaccines.

- The FDA demands warning labels and safety limits for aluminum in intravenous feeding solutions but requires no warnings or safety limits for aluminum in vaccines.

38.

Autism may be related to genetic factors and aluminum-containing pediatric vaccines

"Evidence has now emerged showing that autism may in part result from early-life immune insults induced by environmental xenobiotics. One of the most common xenobiotic with immuno-stimulating as well as neurotoxic properties to which infants under two years of age are routinely exposed worldwide is the aluminum vaccine adjuvant."

Shaw CA, Sheth S, et al. **Etiology of autism spectrum disorders: genes, environment, or both?** *OA Autism* 2014 Jun 10; 2(2): 11.

- This paper reviewed the scientific literature on the immunological and neurological adverse effects of aluminum, especially aluminum adjuvants in vaccines, and its plausible role in autism.

- Although the etiology of autism is related to genetic factors, evidence indicates that early-life assaults to the immune system induced by environmental factors such as aluminum-containing vaccines, must be considered as well.

- Aluminum adjuvants in vaccines stimulate the immune system to produce high antibody levels but they can also provoke serious autoimmune and inflammatory adverse reactions.

- Vaccines with aluminum adjuvants are injected into the body bypassing the protective barriers of the gastrointestinal tract and skin. Absorption of aluminum by this mode is more efficient than through ingestion, increasing the likelihood of a toxic outcome.

- Vaccine-derived aluminum can a) persist in the body for long periods, b) trigger pathological immune responses, c) damage the central nervous system, and d) alter the expression of genes affecting inflammatory processes.

- Children worldwide are exposed to greater quantities of aluminum-containing vaccines than adults.

- Genetic predispositions may sensitize some children to central nervous system damage induced by aluminum-containing pediatric vaccines.

39.

Aluminum in vaccines can provoke permanent malfunctions of the brain and immune system

"Because children may be most at risk of vaccine-induced complications, a rigorous evaluation of the vaccine-related adverse health impacts in the pediatric population is urgently needed."

Tomljenovic L, Shaw CA. **Mechanisms of aluminum adjuvant toxicity and autoimmunity in pediatric populations.** *Lupus* 2012; 21(2): 223-30.

- This paper analyzed the effects of aluminum adjuvant toxicity from vaccines on the developing child's neurological and immune systems.

- Although aluminum is a neurotoxin, preschool children are repeatedly injected with high quantities of aluminum adjuvants from multiple vaccines during critical periods of brain development. This may lead to neurodevelopmental and autoimmune disorders.

- During postnatal development, the child's brain is more permeable to toxins and the kidneys are less able to eliminate them. Thus, children have a greater risk than adults of adverse reactions to aluminum adjuvants in vaccines.

- The same processes that cause aluminum adjuvants to boost immunity can induce immune hyperactivity, a known risk for autoimmune diseases.

- Genetic resistance to autoimmunity can be overridden following concurrent administration of just two or three immune adjuvants.

- The immune stimulating properties of aluminum adjuvants in vaccines have similarities with several autoimmune/inflammatory diseases, such as arthritis, multiple sclerosis, type 1 diabetes, inflammatory bowel disease, chronic fatigue syndrome, lupus, and autism spectrum disorders.

- Vaccine safety studies will often compare an aluminum-containing vaccine to an aluminum adjuvant "placebo," a practice that yields false data on vaccine-related adverse reactions.

40.

Aluminum in vaccines can cause chronic fatigue, sleep disturbances, multiple sclerosis-like demyelinating disorders, and memory problems

"On the grounds of our clinical and experimental data, we believe that increased attention should be paid to possible long-term neurologic effects of continuously escalating doses of alum-containing vaccines administered to the general population."

Gherardi RK, Authier F. **Macrophagic myofasciitis: characterization and pathophysiology**. *Lupus* 2012 Feb; 21(2): 184-89.

- This paper summarizes the evidence on macrophagic myofasciitis (MMF), a disabling health condition that occurs in some people after receiving an aluminum-containing vaccine.

- Aluminum in vaccines may collect at the site of injection or circulate in the blood, travel to other cells and lymph nodes, and eventually accumulate in distant organs such as the spleen and brain.

- Most patients with MMF have an aluminum-filled lesion in the muscle at the site of a previous vaccination.

- Symptoms of MMF include chronic fatigue, chronic diffuse myalgia (muscle weakness), arthralgia (joint pain), cognitive dysfunctions affecting memory and attention, sleep disturbances, and disabling headaches.

- Nearly 20% of patients with MMF develop an autoimmune disease, including neuromuscular and multiple sclerosis-like demyelinating disorders.

- MMF can be induced in mice, rats and monkeys by vaccinating them.

- MMF and autoimmune syndrome induced by adjuvants (ASIA) are similar ailments.

41.

Chronic fatigue, chronic pain, and cognitive disorders have all been linked to aluminum in vaccines

"Macrophagic myofasciitis (MMF) lesions correspond to long-lasting aluminic granulomas, resulting from previous intramuscular injection of aluminum-adjuvanted vaccines."

Rigolet M, Aouizerate J, et al. **Clinical features in patients with long-lasting macrophagic myofasciitis.** *Front Neurol* 2014 Nov 28; 5: 230.

- Macrophagic myofasciitis (MMF) is characterized by aluminum hydroxide muscle lesions at the site of an earlier vaccination. The lesions are persistent, long-term granulomas found in the deltoid muscles of adults and quadriceps in children, common vaccination sites.

- Several vaccines contain aluminum hydroxide, which has been identified as the causal factor of MMF lesions.

- Adult patients with persistent MMF lesions often develop chronic musculoskeletal pain (arthromyalgias), chronic fatigue, and cognitive disorders (including memory impairment and dysexecutive syndrome). Mood disorders, headache, and shortness of breath are common symptoms as well.

- Women are more likely than men to develop MMF.

- The average time between the onset of MMF symptoms and diagnosis is 5.5 years, although the condition is most likely under-diagnosed.

- Autoimmune/inflammatory syndrome induced by adjuvants (ASIA) is another term for a similar set of common symptoms.

42.

Aluminum in vaccines can cause macrophagic myofasciitis, chronic fatigue, and muscle weakness

"Macrophagic myofaciitis may be defined as an emerging novel condition that may be triggered by exposure to alum-containing vaccines, in patients with a specific genetic background."

Israeli E, Agmon-Levin N, et al. **Macrophagic myofaciitis a vaccine (alum) autoimmune-related disease.** *Clin Rev Allergy Immu* 2011 Oct; 41(2): 163-8.

- Aluminum in vaccines can cause macrophagic myofaciitis (MMF), an adverse immune reaction that manifests as chronic fatigue, myalgia, arthralgia, and muscle weakness.
- MMF is accompanied by an immunologically active lesion in the muscle where the aluminum-containing vaccine was injected.

43.

Exley C, Swarbrick L, et al. **A role for the body burden of aluminium in vaccine-associated macrophagic myofasciitis and chronic fatigue syndrome.** *Med Hypotheses* 2009 Feb; 72(2): 135-39.

"Macrophagic myofasciitis and chronic fatigue syndrome are severely disabling conditions which may be caused by adverse reactions to aluminium-containing adjuvants in vaccines."

44.

Lach B, Cupler EJ. **Macrophagic myofasciitis in children is a localized reaction to vaccination.** *J Child Neurol* 2008 Jun; 23(6): 614-19.

"We believe that macrophagic myofasciitis represents a localized histological hallmark of previous immunization with the aluminum hydroxide adjuvants contained in vaccines, rather than a primary or distinct inflammatory muscle disease."

45.

Aluminum in vaccines can cause central nervous system disorders and multiple sclerosis-like symptoms

"The association between macrophagic myofasciitis (MMF) and multiple sclerosis-like disorders may give new insights into the controversial issues surrounding vaccinations and demyelinating central nervous system disorders."

Authier FJ, Cherin P, et al. **Central nervous system disease in patients with macrophagic myofasciitis.** *Brain* 2001 May; 124(Pt 5): 974-83.

- MMF manifests as diffuse myalgia (muscle pain) and multiple sclerosis-like demyelinating central nervous system disorders. It occurs following a persistent local reaction to injections of aluminum-containing vaccines.
- A muscle biopsy and diagnosis of MMF can occur between 3 months and more than 6 years following receipt of an aluminum-containing vaccine.

46.

Gherardi RK, Coquet M, et al. **Macrophagic myofasciitis lesions assess long-term persistence of vaccine-derived aluminium hydroxide in muscle.** *Brain* 2001 Sep; 124(Pt 9): 1821-31.

"We conclude that the MMF lesion is secondary to intramuscular injection of aluminium hydroxide-containing vaccines, shows both long-term persistence of aluminium hydroxide and an ongoing local immune reaction, and is detected in patients with systemic symptoms which appeared subsequently to vaccination."

- Blood tests of patients with macrophagic myofasciitis revealed exposure to vaccines containing an immune stimulating aluminum adjuvant.
- Diffuse myalgia and fatigue were significantly more frequent in patients with, rather than without, a MMF lesion in the deltoid muscle where an aluminum-containing vaccine was injected.

47.

Aluminum in vaccines can travel to distant organs, like the spleen and brain, and become "insidiously unsafe"

"Alum has high neurotoxic potential, and administration of continuously escalating doses of this poorly biodegradable adjuvant in the population should be carefully evaluated by regulatory agencies since the compound may be insidiously unsafe."

Khan Z, Combadière C, et al. **Slow CCL2-dependent translocation of biopersistent particles from muscle to brain.** *BMC Med* 2013; 11: 99.

- Scientists designed several mouse experiments to determine the biological distribution of vaccine-related aluminum.
- Aluminum in vaccines travels from the injection site to distant organs such as the spleen and brain, where it was still detected one year later.
- Aluminum remains in cells long after vaccination and can cause neurologic disorders and autoimmune syndrome induced by adjuvants (ASIA).

48.

Shaw CA, Li Y, Tomljenovic L. **Administration of aluminium to neonatal mice in vaccine-relevant amounts is associated with adverse long term neurological outcomes.** *J Inorg Biochem* 2013 Nov; 128: 237-44.

"These current data implicate aluminum injected in early postnatal life in some central nervous system alterations that may be relevant for a better understanding of the etiology of autism spectrum disorders."

- In this study, young mice were injected with either high or low levels of aluminum adjuvants (designed to correlate with U.S. or Scandinavian childhood vaccine schedules).
- Significant changes in the mice were observed, affirming the role of aluminum adjuvants in adversely altering the central nervous system.

49.

Aluminum adjuvants added to vaccines are "insidiously unsafe" and may cause long-term cognitive deficits

"Studies on animal models and humans have shown that aluminum adjuvants by themselves cause autoimmune and inflammatory conditions. These findings plausibly implicate aluminum adjuvants in pediatric vaccines as causal factors contributing to increased rates of autism spectrum disorders in countries where multiple doses are almost universally administered."

Shaw CA, Seneff S, et al. **Aluminum-induced entropy in biological systems: implications for neurological disease.** *J Toxicol* 2014; 2014: 491316.

- Aluminum exposure produces adverse effects in living organisms and is especially damaging to the central nervous system. It is unsafe even in trace quantities.

- This paper provides extensive evidence that aluminum exposure in all of the forms studied, including aluminum administered as an immune-stimulating adjuvant added to vaccines, is harmful.

- Aluminum hydroxide, a common vaccine adjuvant, is "insidiously unsafe." Cumulative doses of aluminum from vaccines can induce long-term cognitive deficits such as encephalopathy and degenerative dementia.

- Aluminum from vaccine adjuvants crosses the blood-brain and blood-cerebrospinal fluid barriers, provoking harmful immuno-inflammatory responses in neural tissues.

- Clinical studies on vaccine safety often administer aluminum-containing injections to a "control" group as a harmless "placebo" despite evidence that aluminum is toxic to humans and animals. Its use as a placebo cannot be justified.

50.

Aluminum in vaccines can cause neuron death plus motor and memory deficits similar to Gulf War Syndrome

"The demonstrated neurotoxicity of aluminum hydroxide and its relative ubiquity as an adjuvant suggest that greater scrutiny by the scientific community is warranted."

Shaw CA, Petrik MS. **Aluminum hydroxide injections lead to motor deficits and motor neuron degeneration.** *J Inorg Biochem* 2009 Nov; 103(11): 1555.

- Gulf War Syndrome afflicted many veterans of Western militaries with cognitive and motor deficits similar to amyotrophic lateral sclerosis (ALS), a progressive neurodegenerative disease that destroys nerve cells.
- This study looked at whether aluminum (and squalene) adjuvants in vaccines given to Gulf War vets could be linked to cognitive and behavioral deficits.
- Aluminum-injected mice showed significant deficits in memory and motor functions. They also had pathological abnormalities that are characteristic of neurological diseases such as Alzheimer's and dementia.
- The results reported in this paper correspond with other studies demonstrating that aluminum adjuvants can be neurotoxic.

51.

Petrik MS, Wong MC, et al. **Aluminum adjuvant linked to Gulf War illness induces motor neuron death in mice.** *Neuromolecular Med* 2007; 9(1): 83-100.

"These findings suggest a possible role for the aluminum adjuvant in some neurological features associated with Gulf War Illness."

- In this study, mice were injected with adjuvants at doses equivalent to those given to vaccinated U.S. Gulf War veterans. Testing showed significant motor neuron loss and progressive deficits in strength.

52.

Aluminum in vaccines can cause cognitive dysfunction, chronic fatigue, autoimmunity, and Gulf War syndrome

"Long-term persistence of vaccine-derived aluminum hydroxide within the body...is associated with cognitive dysfunction."

Couette M, Boisse MF, et al. **Long-term persistence of vaccine-derived aluminum hydroxide is associated with chronic cognitive dysfunction.** *J Inorg Biochem* 2009 Nov; 103(11): 1571-78.

- Researchers designed neuropsychological tests to assess cognitive dysfunction in patients who developed macrophagic myofasciitis from vaccines containing aluminum hydroxide.
- Cognitive dysfunction associated with macrophagic myofasciitis mainly affects executive functions such as memory, attention and planning.

53.

Gherardi RK. **Lessons from macrophagic myofasciitis: towards definition of a vaccine adjuvant-related syndrome**. *Rev Neurol (Paris)* 2003 Feb; 159(2): 162-64.

- Macrophagic myofasciitis is recognized by an immunologically active lesion that can persist for years in the deltoid muscle at the site of a vaccine injection containing an aluminum adjuvant.
- Symptoms of vaccine-induced macrophagic myofasciitis include myalgias and chronic fatigue in half of patients, and autoimmune disease such as multiple sclerosis in one-third of cases. Chronic immune stimulation can also cause rheumatoid arthritis.
- Many Gulf war veterans have symptoms similar to patients with macrophagic myofasciitis. Multiple vaccinations administered over a short time period have been recognized as the main risk factor for Gulf War syndrome.

54.

Aluminum-adjuvant vaccines can damage the nervous system and cause autoimmune disorders

"Aluminum has been demonstrated to impact the central nervous system at every level, including by changing gene expression. These outcomes should raise concerns about the increasing use of aluminum salts as vaccine adjuvants."

Shaw CA, Li D, Tomljenovic L. **Are there negative CNS impacts of aluminum adjuvants used in vaccines and immunotherapy?** *Immunotherapy* 2014; 6(10): 1055-71.

- This paper reviewed the scientific literature on the use of aluminum salts as vaccine adjuvants, including their toxic effects on the nervous system and the potential to induce autoimmunity.
- Aluminum-adjuvant vaccines can cause macrophagic myofasciitis (MMF). Clinical symptoms include myalgia, arthralgia, chronic fatigue, autoimmunity, and cognitive dysfunction.
- Although MMF is associated with a macrophagic lesion at the site of vaccination, it is a systemic ailment.
- MMF patients are usually middle-aged women who received at least one aluminum-containing vaccine in the 10 years prior to MMF diagnosis.
- Aluminum-adjuvant vaccines can cause ASIA syndrome, associated with autoimmune disorders.
- In Western nations, children may be injected with 4.225 mg of aluminum during infancy and up to 1.475 mg of aluminum during a single pediatric visit.
- Nations that require the most aluminum-adjuvant vaccines for children have the highest autism rates.
- Based on the current scientific literature, it is unlikely that in the future aluminum will be considered safe for use in vaccines.

55.

Aluminum adjuvants in vaccines can be dangerous, causing autoimmunity and ASIA syndrome in some people

"Experimental research has shown that aluminum adjuvants have a potential to induce serious immunological disorders in humans."

Perricone C, Colafrancesco S, et al. **Autoimmune/inflammatory syndrome induced by adjuvants (ASIA) 2013: Unveiling the pathogenic, clinical and diagnostic aspects.** *J Autoimmun* 2013 Dec; 47: 1-16.

- Many vaccines contain aluminum adjuvants to stimulate an immune response. In susceptible individuals, these vaccines can cause ASIA syndrome, an autoimmune disease with neurological and cognitive manifestations.

- Aluminum adjuvants in vaccines have also been linked to conditions such as arthritis, multiple sclerosis, systemic lupus erythematosus, chronic fatigue syndrome, Gulf War syndrome, macrophagic myofasciitis, granuloma formation and allergic reactions.

- Clinical symptoms associated with vaccine-induced autoimmunity can take months or years to manifest, much longer than the time intervals utilized in most vaccine safety studies.

- Genetic differences can cause people to react differently to vaccines. Therefore, vaccination schedules should be personalized and scientists should develop predictive techniques to determine which populations are more likely to have adverse reactions to vaccines.

56.

Vaccine adjuvants such as aluminum and oil-in-water emulsions may cause autoimmune diseases

"The idea that the adjuvant component of vaccines could enhance or trigger autoimmunity or autoimmune diseases represents an intriguing observation that may explain a number of adverse reactions observed after vaccination."

Pellegrino P, Clementi E, Radice S. **On vaccine's adjuvants and autoimmunity: current evidence and future perspectives.** *Autoimmun Rev* 2015 Oct; 14(10): 880-88.

- In this paper, researchers reviewed the scientific literature on the use of adjuvants in vaccines, including the ways in which they may induce autoimmune adverse reactions.
- Adjuvants are substances added to vaccines to improve the immune response. They may conserve antigen doses while increasing antibody titers.
- Several adjuvants exist, each with specific mechanisms of action that could alter the immune response and risk of adverse effects.
- Currently approved adjuvants include aluminum salts, oil-in-water emulsions (MF59, AS03 and AF03), virosomes and AS04.
- MF59 contains squalene. AS03 contains squalene and α-tocopherol, which has been linked to the development of narcolepsy, a chronic sleeping disorder.
- Adjuvants can cause ASIA syndrome, a spectrum of immune damage and debilitating post-vaccination adverse reactions.
- Several factors can influence immune response and the risk of adverse events after vaccination, including genetic predisposition, concomitant drugs, race and gender.

57.

Mercury and aluminum in vaccines can cause autoimmunity and neurological disorders

"The present study represents the first clear-cut meta-analysis of a molecular platform able to rationalize the potential cause-effect link between vaccination and subsequent adverse events."

Kanduc D. **Peptide cross-reactivity: the original sin of vaccines.** *Front Biosci (Schol Ed)* 2012 Jun 1; 4: 1393-1401.

- This paper describes several problems with current vaccine technology, such as the ability of microbes to evade the immune system, and the use of adjuvants which can cause autoimmunity.
- Vaccines based on antigens from infectious matter induce a poor or non-existent immune response. This is why adjuvants such as aluminum hydroxide and oil emulsions are included in vaccines to stimulate immune responses.
- Adjuvants can induce hyperactivation of the immune system, initiating auto-immune processes. Autoimmune attacks against myelin may cause demyelinating diseases, while attacks against proteins and antigens affecting cognition and behavior may cause autism and behavior disorders.

58.

Dórea JG. **Exposure to mercury and aluminum in early life: developmental vulnerability as a modifying factor in neurologic and immunologic effects.** *Int J Environ Res Public Health* 2015 Jan 23; 12(2): 1295-13.

- This paper reviewed the scientific literature on the effects of mercury and aluminum in vaccines on newborns and infants.
- Mercury and aluminum affect neurologic, immunologic, and renal systems.
- The synergistic effect of mercury and aluminum, toxic agents in some vaccines, has not been properly studied.

59.

Repeatedly vaccinated sheep and mice developed autoimmune injuries

"The present report is the first description of a new sheep syndrome (ovine ASIA syndrome) linked to multiple, repetitive vaccination and that can have devastating consequences as it happened after the compulsory vaccination against bluetongue in 2008."

Luján L, Pérez M, et al. **Autoimmune/autoinflammatory syndrome induced by adjuvants (ASIA syndrome) in commercial sheep.** *Immunol Res* 2013 Jul; 56(2-3): 317-24.

- This paper identifies a new form of autoimmune/inflammatory syndrome induced by adjuvants (ASIA syndrome) in sheep, linked to vaccinations containing aluminum adjuvants.

- The condition appears in some sheep 2-6 days after they are vaccinated. Symptoms of the acute phase include poor response to external stimuli and acute meningoencephalitis. The chronic phase causes muscular atrophy, neurodegeneration of the gray matter of the spinal cord, and death.

60.

Tsumiyama K, Miyazaki Y, Shiozawa S. **Self-organized criticality theory of autoimmunity.** *PLoS ONE* 2009; 4(12): e8382.

"Autoimmunity appears to be the inevitable consequence of overstimulating the host's immune system by repeated immunization."

- Scientists repeatedly vaccinated mice that are not prone to autoimmune diseases. They found that overstimulation of the immune system eventually results in autoimmune injury similar to systemic lupus erythematosus.

- T cells in repeatedly-vaccinated mice eventually produced autoantibodies.

- Systemic autoimmunity occurs when a host's T cells are overstimulated by repeated exposure to antigens beyond the integrity of their immune systems.

61.

Some people may be predisposed to developing vaccine-induced autoimmunity

"Historically, vaccine trials have routinely excluded vulnerable individuals with a variety of pre-existing conditions. Because of such selection bias, the occurrence of serious adverse reactions resulting from vaccinations in real life where vaccines are mandated to all individuals regardless of their susceptibility factors may be considerably underestimated."

Soriano A, Nesher G, Shoenfeld Y. **Predicting post-vaccination autoimmunity: who might be at risk?** *Pharmacol Res* 2015 Feb; 92: 18-22.

- This paper reviewed the scientific literature to assess who might be at increased risk of developing a vaccine-induced autoimmune disease.

- People with a previous history of vaccine-related adverse reactions, a family history of autoimmune diseases, the presence of auto-antibodies or certain genetic signatures, may be more susceptible to developing autoimmunity following vaccinations.

- Adverse reactions and autoimmune ailments such as ASIA syndrome may be triggered by vaccine ingredients, including aluminum adjuvants.

- Potential autoimmune diseases following vaccinations include systemic lupus erythematosus, arthritis, diabetes, thrombocytopenia, vasculitis, Guillain-Barré syndrome and demyelinating disorders.

- Nearly all vaccines have been associated with autoimmune conditions. A link between autoimmunity and a previous vaccine is not always apparent.

Influenza

The influenza vaccine was originally developed in the 1940s to protect military personnel. In 1960, influenza vaccines were recommended for adults over 65 years of age. Today, they are strongly encouraged or mandated for nearly everyone, including infants over the age of 6 months, children, teens, pregnant women (all trimesters), healthy adults, the elderly, and healthcare workers. About 170 million doses were expected to be produced for the U.S. market alone during the 2015/2016 influenza season, a substantial increase over the 32 million doses made available in 1990.

The scientific papers in this chapter document several problems with influenza vaccines. For example, studies show that annual vaccination against seasonal influenza reduces protective immunity against more virulent pandemic strains. People who are naturally exposed to circulating influenza viruses — unvaccinated individuals — are likely to gain cross-protection against other strains of the disease. Vaccinated people are denied this cross-protective benefit. Animal studies confirm the health benefits of prior infection. Mice that were infected with a non-lethal strain of influenza and then exposed to a lethal strain had a better survival rate than mice that were not infected prior to being exposed to a lethal strain.

Other scientific papers show that the CDC policy of vaccinating pregnant women is not supported by science, the influenza vaccine is not very effective, and children who receive an inactivated influenza vaccine are significantly more likely than non-vaccinated children to be hospitalized. Although influenza vaccines were originally recommended for the elderly, there is no evidence that influenza vaccines improve elderly death rates. There is also no evidence that vaccinating healthcare workers protects their patients.

Influenza vaccine marketing campaigns are also problematic. Health authorities and the CDC use scare tactics, exaggerate the dangers of influenza and inflate the benefits of influenza vaccination to increase the number of people who receive influenza vaccines. These unethical practices restrict the possibilities for rational discussion and reasonable public health policy.

62.

Annual vaccination against common strains of influenza reduces protective immunity against more dangerous strains of the disease

"Since young children are immunologically naive to influenza viruses, vaccination of this age group every year might prevent the induction of heterosubtypic immunity, leaving infants more susceptible to pandemic strains of influenza."

Bodewes R, Kreijtz JH, Rimmelzwaan GF. **Yearly influenza vaccinations: a double-edged sword?** *Lancet Infect Dis* 2009 Dec; 9(12): 784-88.

- Many countries recommend annual influenza vaccinations for members of their population. This paper assessed the wisdom of this practice.

- Natural infection with common influenza A viruses provides heterosubtypic immunity, that is, protection against more lethal influenza A viruses of other unrelated subtypes.

- Vaccination against seasonal influenza interferes with the development of natural protective immunity against potentially lethal infections from new subtypes of the influenza virus.

- Annual vaccinations of young children against common influenza strains could be counterproductive, preventing them from acquiring more comprehensive immunity, leaving them unprotected against dangerous pandemic strains of the disease.

- Studies conducted on mice show that heterosubtypic immunity is essential to staying alive.

- The recommendation in several countries to vaccinate all healthy children 6-59 months of age against influenza should be reassessed because it could interfere with protection against newly emerging and more virulent influenza A virus subtypes.

63.

Prior vaccination against seasonal influenza may increase the risk of contracting a severe case of pandemic influenza

"We report findings from four epidemiologic studies in Canada showing that prior receipt of 2008-09 trivalent inactivated influenza vaccine was associated with increased risk of medically attended pandemic H1N1 illness during the spring-summer 2009."

Skowronski DM, De Serres G, et al. **Association between the 2008–09 seasonal influenza vaccine and pandemic H1N1 illness during Spring–Summer 2009: four observational studies from Canada.** *PLoS Med* 2010 April 6; 7(4): e1000258.

- Four studies showed that recipients of a seasonal influenza vaccine had a significantly increased risk of subsequently developing severe pandemic influenza compared to people who did not receive the seasonal vaccine.
- Prior receipt of a seasonal influenza vaccine significantly increased the risk of requiring medical attention for illness due to the novel H1N1 pandemic influenza virus (odds ratio, OR = 1.4 to 2.5).
- Annual vaccination against seasonal influenza may prevent the more robust, complex, and cross-protective immunity gained by natural infection.
- These findings have scientific implications about the relationship between seasonal and pandemic influenza strains, and how to control influenza.

64.

Crum-Cianflone NF, Blair PJ, et al. **Clinical and epidemiologic characteristics of an outbreak of novel H1N1 (swine origin) influenza A virus among United States military beneficiaries.** *Clin Infect Dis* 2009 Dec 15; 49(12): 1801-10.

- Active duty members of the military infected with novel H1N1 pandemic influenza (swine flu) were significantly more likely than those without pandemic influenza virus infection to have received a seasonal influenza shot.

65.

Mice that were infected with a seasonal influenza virus survived exposure to a lethal influenza strain; vaccinated mice died

"During a next pandemic, especially children that received the annual flu-shot would be at higher risk to develop severe illness and a fatal outcome of the disease than those that experienced an infection with a seasonal influenza A virus strain. This of course would be of great concern and is supported by the data obtained in our mouse model."

Bodewes R, Kreijtz JH, et al. **Vaccination against human influenza A/H3N2 virus prevents the induction of heterosubtypic immunity against lethal infection with Avian influenza A/H5N1 virus.** *PloS One* 2009; 4(5): e5538.

- Natural infection with seasonal strains of influenza provides heterosubtypic immunity (cross-protection) against more virulent pandemic strains of a different subtype.

- Cell-mediated immunity induced by natural infection with seasonal influenza viruses usually causes a non-severe upper respiratory tract infection, then confers protection against more virulent pandemic influenza strains.

- Vaccination against moderate seasonal influenza strains prevents cross protection against lethal influenza strains.

- Mice that were vaccinated against a seasonal influenza virus and then infected with a virulent pandemic avian influenza virus had lung virus titers on day 7 post-infection that were 100 times higher than mice that were not vaccinated against seasonal influenza prior to infection with pandemic influenza.

- The vaccinated mice had more severe disease and died when exposed to pandemic influenza. The unvaccinated mice survived.

- The findings in this study encourage reconsideration of the standard recommendation to vaccinate all healthy children against seasonal influenza.

66.

Mice vaccinated against seasonal influenza died after exposure to pandemic influenza; unvaccinated mice survived

"Annual vaccination may hamper the development of cross-reactive immunity against influenza A viruses of novel subtypes, that would otherwise be induced by natural infection."

Bodewes R, Fraaij PL, et al. **Annual influenza vaccination affects the development of heterosubtypic immunity.** *Vaccine* 2012 Dec 7; 30(51): 7407-10.

- This paper summarizes earlier studies on cross-protective immunity in mice.

67.

Kreijtz JH, Bodewes R, et al. **Infection of mice with a human influenza A/H3N2 virus induces protective immunity against lethal infection with influenza A/H5N1 virus.** *Vaccine* 2009 Aug 6; 27(36): 4983-89.

- Mice were infected with a non-lethal influenza virus and then exposed to a lethal strain 4 weeks later. Other mice were not infected with a non-lethal influenza virus prior to being exposed to the lethal strain. The infected mice had fewer clinical symptoms and less mortality than the uninfected mice.

- Prior infections with seasonal influenza viruses confer protection against more virulent influenza strains. Pre-existing heterosubtypic immunity could lessen the impact of a future influenza pandemic.

68.

Kreijtz JH, Bodewes R, et al. **Primary influenza A virus infection induces cross-protective immunity against a lethal infection with a heterosubtypic virus strain in mice.** *Vaccine* 2007 Jan 8; 25(4): 612-20.

- Mice infected with a non-lethal influenza virus were then exposed to a lethal strain. They cleared the infection more quickly and had a better survival rate than mice that were not infected prior to being exposed to the lethal strain.

69.

The current season's influenza vaccine will not work in people who also received the previous season's influenza vaccine

"In vaccinated subjects with no evidence of prior season vaccination, significant protection (62%) against community-acquired influenza was demonstrated. Substantially lower effectiveness was noted among subjects who were vaccinated in both the current and prior season."

Ohmit SE, Petrie JG, et al. **Influenza vaccine effectiveness in the community and the household.** *Clin Infect Dis* 2013 May; 56(10): 1363-69.

- In this study, 328 families with 1441 household members (60% vaccinated/ 40% unvaccinated) were followed through an entire influenza season.
- Both vaccinated and unvaccinated people contracted laboratory-confirmed influenza at similar rates. The vaccine provided no significant protection.
- The only people who benefitted from an influenza vaccine during the influenza season were those who did not also receive an influenza vaccine during the previous season.
- People who had been vaccinated 2 years in a row were not protected against influenza. In fact, vaccine effectiveness was -45% (negative 45 percent).
- Adults who were vaccinated 2 years in a row were just as likely to contract influenza as adults who were not vaccinated in either year.
- The vaccine did not protect family members who were exposed to influenza in their own homes. In fact, 82% of adults who contracted influenza from another member of the family were vaccinated. The vaccine effectiveness in this group was -51% (negative 51 percent).

70.

Pregnant women vaccinated against seasonal influenza and A-H1N1 (swine flu) had high rates of spontaneous abortions

"Just because a single vaccine has been tested and considered safe does not imply there will not be a synergistic fetal toxicity effect associated with the administration of two or more Thimerosal-containing vaccines to a pregnant women and/or a synergistic toxicity effect from the combination of the biologically active components contained in concomitantly administered vaccines."

Goldman GS. **Comparison of VAERS fetal-loss reports during three consecutive influenza seasons: Was there a synergistic fetal toxicity associated with the two-vaccine 2009/2010 season?** *Hum Exp Toxicol* 2013 May; 32(5): 464-75.

- The CDC recommends influenza vaccines for pregnant women. However, some women lose their babies after receiving an influenza vaccine.

- This study compared the number of fetal losses reported to the government during influenza seasons when pregnant women received one influenza vaccine versus the 2009/2010 influenza season when pregnant women received two influenza vaccines — a seasonal shot and the A-H1N1 "swine flu" vaccine.

- Prior to vaccinating pregnant women against seasonal influenza and swine flu during the 2009/2010 influenza season, the swine flu shot was never tested for safety (or efficacy) in pregnant women. Nor were two different influenza vaccines ever co-administered and tested for safety in pregnant women.

- Both the seasonal and swine flu vaccines contained 25 mcg of mercury per dose, exceeding EPA safety levels by several thousand-fold for an early developing fetus during the first trimester.

- There were 77.8 fetal loss reports per 1 million pregnant women vaccinated during the 2009/2010 2-dose influenza season vs. 6.8 fetal loss reports per 1 million pregnant women vaccinated during the previous 1-dose influenza season — a highly statistically significant 11.4-fold increase.

71.

CDC policy to vaccinate pregnant women with thimerosal-containing influenza vaccines is not supported by science

"The [CDC] recommendation of influenza vaccination during pregnancy is not supported by citations in its own policy paper or in current medical literature. Considering the potential risks of maternal and fetal mercury exposure, the administration of thimerosal during pregnancy is both unjustified and unwise."

Ayoub DM, Yazbak FE. **Influenza vaccination during pregnancy: a critical assessment of the recommendations of the Advisory Committee on Immunization Practices (ACIP).** *Journal of American Physicians and Surgeons* 2006 Summer; 11(2): 41-47.

- The CDC's Advisory Committee on Immunization Practices (ACIP) recommends influenza vaccination during all trimesters of pregnancy. This paper critically reviewed this policy and the citations used to justify it.

- The CDC cites only two papers to support its claim that influenza is more dangerous during pregnancy. Both papers failed to show that influenza during pregnancy is more serious than at other times.

- CDC estimates on vaccine efficacy are not supported by the scientific literature. In a large study utilizing the CDC's own database — the Vaccine Safety Datalink — there were no significant differences in illness rates among vaccinated and unvaccinated pregnant women or their children.

- In another study, vaccinated pregnant women were 4 times more likely to be hospitalized for influenza-like illness than unvaccinated pregnant women.

- Most influenza vaccines for pregnant women contain 25 mcg of mercury, a quantity that greatly exceeds EPA safety limits. The vaccine manufacturer's Safety Data Sheet discusses thimerosal: "Exposure in utero can cause mild to severe mental retardation and motor coordination impairment."

- The CDC's policy of recommending influenza vaccination to pregnant women is not supported by scientific data and should be discontinued.

72.

The influenza vaccine is not very effective, causes adverse reactions, and can spread disease to other people

"The yearly U.S. mass influenza vaccination campaign has been ineffective in preventing influenza in vaccine recipients. Vaccine recipients need to be informed of the limitations and risks of the vaccine and of the alternatives to vaccination. In particular, they need to know of the possibility that repeated vaccinations may increase the risk of adverse effects."

Geier DA, King PG, et al. **Influenza vaccine: review of effectiveness of the U.S. immunization program, and policy considerations.** *Journal of American Physicians and Surgeons* 2006 Fall; 11(3): 69-74.

- This study analyzed 18 years of data and concluded that the influenza vaccine has little or no effectiveness over the U.S. population for preventing influenza cases, hospital admissions, or deaths.

- People who receive live virus influenza vaccines are at risk of adverse reactions and can also transmit the disease to people they come in contact with, including pregnant women and those with weak immunity.

- Recipients of live virus influenza vaccines are warned to avoid close contact with immunocompromised people for 3 weeks.

- Live virus influenza vaccines could potentially cause a "super virus" if the vaccine strain recombines with another viral infection contracted by the vaccinated person.

- About 1,300 Americans die every year from influenza, considerably less than the unsubstantiated 36,000 deaths often claimed by health authorities.

73.

Influenza vaccines are not effective in young children; safety data can't be trusted

"The manufacturers' refusal to release all safety outcome data from trials carried out in young children, together with obvious reporting bias and inconsistencies in the primary studies does not bode well for a fair assessment of the safety of live attenuated vaccines."

Jefferson T, Rivetti A, et al. **Vaccines for preventing influenza in healthy children.** *Cochrane Database Syst Rev* 2012 Aug 15; Issue 8: CD004879.

- This review analyzed all relevant influenza vaccine studies — 75 studies from around the world, including 17 randomized controlled trials — to evaluate the effects of influenza vaccines in healthy children.
- In children older than two years of age, the live influenza vaccine is about 33% effective (RR = 0.67); inactivated influenza vaccines are about 36% effective (RR = 0.64).
- In children under two years of age, inactivated influenza vaccines "have similar effects to placebo."
- No convincing evidence could be found showing that influenza vaccines can reduce mortality, hospital admissions, serious complications or community transmission of influenza.

74.

Jefferson T, Smith S, et al. **Assessment of the efficacy and effectiveness of influenza vaccines in healthy children: systematic review.** *Lancet* 2005 Feb 26; 365(9461): 773-80.

"We recorded no convincing evidence that vaccines can reduce mortality, admissions, serious complications, and community transmission of influenza."

- The findings in this paper do not support vaccinating very young children against influenza.

75.

Children who receive an inactivated influenza vaccine are significantly more likely than non-vaccinated children to be hospitalized

"Trivalent inactivated influenza vaccine did not provide any protection against hospitalization in pediatric subjects, especially children with asthma. On the contrary, we found a threefold increased risk of hospitalization in subjects who did get trivalent inactivated influenza vaccine."

Joshi AY, Iyer VN, et al. **Effectiveness of trivalent inactivated influenza vaccine in influenza-related hospitalization in children: a case-control study.** *Allergy Asthma Proc* 2012 Mar-Apr; 33(2): e23-7.

- Researchers investigated children, 6 months to 18 years old, who contracted laboratory-confirmed influenza. They determined who was hospitalized for the disease and whether they had previously received an influenza vaccine.

- Children who were vaccinated against influenza were 3 times more likely to be hospitalized for influenza-related complications than children who did not receive an influenza vaccine (OR = 3.67).

- Asthmatic children who received the inactivated influenza vaccine were also significantly more likely to be hospitalized than asthmatic children who did not receive the vaccine. The severity of asthma did not affect the results.

- When children contract influenza, they are more likely to require hospital care if they were previously vaccinated against the disease.

- This study shows that when the inactivated influenza vaccine is given to children as recommended by the CDC, it is not only ineffective at preventing laboratory-confirmed influenza-related hospitalization, it actually increases the risk.

- This study was conducted over 8 influenza seasons, from 1999-2000 through 2006-2007.

76.

Children vaccinated against seasonal influenza are not protected and are more likely than non-vaccinated children to develop respiratory virus infections

"We identified a statistically significant increased risk of non-influenza respiratory virus infection among trivalent inactivated influenza vaccine recipients, including significant increases in the risk of rhinovirus and coxsackie/echovirus infection."

Cowling BJ, Fang VJ, et al. **Increased risk of noninfluenza respiratory virus infections associated with receipt of inactivated influenza vaccine.** *Clin Infect Dis* 2012 June 15; 54(12): 1778-83.

- In a double-blind randomized controlled trial, children aged 6-15 years were either vaccinated against seasonal influenza or received a placebo.

- Although children who received an influenza vaccine had a significantly lower risk of seasonal influenza infection *based on serologic evidence,* there was no statistically significant reduction in *confirmed* seasonal influenza infection when compared to children who received a placebo.

- Children who received the influenza vaccine were 4 times more likely than children who received a placebo to develop acute respiratory illness associated with confirmed *non-influenza* respiratory virus infection (RR = 4.40).

- Influenza vaccine recipients were also significantly more likely than those who received a placebo to develop non-influenza respiratory infections from rhinoviruses, coxsackieviruses and echoviruses (RR = 3.46).

- If children who contract influenza gain non-specific immunity protecting them from other respiratory infections, vaccination would suppress this health benefit, explaining why influenza-vaccinated children have a significantly increased risk of developing acute non-influenza respiratory illness.

77.

Hand-washing and teaching children proper hygiene may be more effective than vaccines at reducing the spread of influenza and other respiratory viruses

"The disparity in effectiveness between the high profile of influenza vaccines and antivirals and the low profile of physical interventions is striking. Public health recommendations are almost completely based on the use of vaccines and antivirals despite a lack of strong evidence."

Jefferson T, Del Mar C, et al. **Physical interventions to interrupt or reduce the spread of respiratory viruses: systematic review.** *BMJ* 2009 Sep 21; 339: b3675.

- Fifty-nine studies were reviewed to find evidence of the effectiveness of public health measures to reduce the spread of respiratory viruses.

- Although vaccines and anti-viral drugs are highly promoted to control the spread of influenza, there is scant evidence supporting their widespread use.

- Physical interventions, such as hand washing and wearing masks, are cheap and highly effective at preventing the spread of respiratory viruses. The spread of severe acute respiratory syndrome (SARS) declined by 55% through frequent hand washing (OR = .45) and by 68% through wearing masks (OR = .32).

- The highest quality randomized trials showed that the spread of respiratory viruses can be prevented by teaching young children proper hygiene.

78.

Jefferson T, Del Mar CB, et al. **Physical interventions to interrupt or reduce the spread of respiratory viruses.** *Cochrane Database Syst Rev* 2011 July 6; (7): CD006207.

- Simple, low-cost, non-invasive interventions such as hand washing, especially around young children, may be more effective than vaccines and anti-viral drugs at preventing the spread of influenza and other respiratory viruses.

79.

Influenza-related death rates in the elderly do not improve by increasing influenza vaccination rates in the elderly

"We could not correlate increasing vaccination coverage after 1980 with declining mortality rates in any age group. We conclude that observational studies substantially overestimate vaccination benefit."

Simonsen L, Reichert TA, et al. **Impact of influenza vaccination on seasonal mortality in the US elderly population.** *Arch Intern Med* 2005 Feb 14; 165(3): 265-72.

- This study analyzed U.S. data from 33 influenza seasons — from 1968 to 2001 — to compare influenza vaccination rates in the elderly and their effect on mortality.

- Prior to 1980, about 15% of elderly persons were vaccinated. By 2001, 65% were vaccinated — a fourfold increase — yet influenza-related mortality rates remained constant.

- Although the influenza vaccination rate in people 65 years or older increased by about 50 percentage points from 1980 to 2001, there was no corresponding decline in influenza-related deaths.

- In 1968, unvaccinated elderly persons were exposed to a pandemic influenza virus. This conferred natural immunity on this population and may be the reason for a decline in influenza-related deaths in the decade that followed.

80.

There is no unbiased scientific evidence that influenza vaccines improve death rates in the elderly

"Cohort studies have consistently reported that vaccination reduces all-cause winter mortality by about 50%—an astonishing claim given that only about 5% of all winter deaths are attributable to influenza. This vaccine efficacy overestimation has now been attributed to profound confounding frailty selection bias."

Simonsen L, Viboud C, et al. **Influenza vaccination and mortality benefits: new insights, new opportunities.** *Vaccine* 2009; 27(45): 6300-4.

- Many countries rely on vaccinating seniors to control influenza. Some studies have reported that this policy is effective and reduces all-cause winter mortality by about 50%, an unbelievable claim since only a small number of winter deaths in seniors are attributed to influenza.
- This paper analyzed the evidence to determine whether mortality rates improve by vaccinating the elderly.
- Excess mortality studies found no decrease in national influenza-related deaths in seniors during a period when vaccination rates in seniors quadrupled.
- During the 1980s and 1990s, the percentage of seniors who received influenza vaccines increased fourfold yet CDC epidemiologists found that national influenza-related death rates actually increased.
- About 75% of all influenza-related deaths occur in people 70 years and older. However, there are no "gold-standard" randomized studies to confirm that influenza vaccines benefit this age group.
- Some studies show that influenza vaccination seemed to prevent mortality more effectively *before* the influenza season even began — unambiguous evidence of selection bias (false randomization).
- Influential medical journals continue to publish studies on influenza vaccine efficacy that contain extensive selection bias.

81.

There is no evidence that vaccinating healthcare workers against influenza to protect their elderly patients is effective

"Vaccinating healthcare workers who care for those aged 60 or over in long-term care institutions showed no effect on laboratory-proven influenza or complications (lower respiratory tract infection, hospitalization or death due to lower respiratory tract illness) in those aged 60 or over resident in long-term care institutions."

Thomas RE, Jefferson T, Lasserson TJ. **Influenza vaccination for healthcare workers who care for people aged 60 or older living in long-term care institutions.** *Cochrane Database Syst Rev* 2013; Issue 7: CD005187.

- Authorities often mandate influenza vaccinations for healthcare workers who may transmit influenza to their elderly patients.
- This paper analyzed all randomized controlled studies where healthcare workers were vaccinated and laboratory tests were then used to determine if their elderly patients were protected against influenza and its complications.
- There is no evidence that vaccinating healthcare workers against influenza prevents laboratory-proven influenza or its complications in their elderly patients living in long-term care institutions.
- There is no evidence to support compulsory influenza vaccination of healthcare workers who care for the elderly in long-term care institutions.

82.

Thomas RE, Jefferson T, Lasserson TJ. **Influenza vaccination for healthcare workers who work with the elderly: systematic review.** *Vaccine* 2010 Dec 16; 29(2): 344-56.

- Pooled data from three randomized controlled studies showed vaccinating healthcare workers against influenza had no effect on influenza, pneumonia, or deaths from pneumonia in their elderly patients.

83.

Healthcare policies that mandate influenza vaccination for healthcare workers to protect their patients are not supported by science

"The studies aiming to prove the widespread belief that staff vaccination has a substantial effect on patient morbidity and mortality are heavily flawed. No reliable evidence shows that healthcare worker vaccination has noteworthy advantage to their patients — not in reducing patient morbidity or mortality, not in increasing patient vaccination, and not in decreasing healthcare worker work absenteeism."

Abramson ZH. **What, in fact, is the evidence that vaccinating healthcare workers against seasonal influenza protects their patients? A critical review.** *Int J Family Med* 2012; 2012: 205464.

- This paper examined all relevant influenza studies to assess the evidence supporting policies that mandate vaccination of healthcare workers to protect their patients.

- Studies cited by health authorities to justify mandating influenza vaccines for all healthcare workers are extremely flawed and such recommendations are biased.

- There is evidence that influenza vaccine study conclusions are manipulated and deceptively promoted.

- There is no evidence that a patient's brief encounter with community clinic healthcare workers substantially increases their risk of contracting influenza.

- There is no reliable evidence that vaccinating healthcare workers against influenza is clearly beneficial to their patients. Such policies are unsound and not supported by the scientific literature.

- Healthcare workers should be free to accept or reject influenza vaccination without being subjected to legal, institutional, or peer coercion.

84.

Influenza vaccine studies have poor quality and their conclusions rarely match the actual data that is in those studies

"Most of our studies (70%) were of poor quality with overoptimistic conclusions — that is, not supported by the data presented. Those sponsored by industry had greater visibility as they were more likely to be published by high impact factor journals and were likely to be given higher prominence by the international scientific and lay media, despite their apparent equivalent methodological quality and size compared with studies with other funders."

Jefferson T, Di Pietrantonj C, et al. **Relation of study quality, concordance, take home message, funding, and impact in studies of influenza vaccines: systematic review.** *BMJ* 2009 Feb 12; 338: b354.

- Researchers analyzed 259 influenza studies to determine a) study quality, b) whether data presented in each study confirmed the authors' conclusions, c) whether the conclusions were supportive or critical of the vaccine being evaluated, and d) whether industry-funded studies receive greater exposure.

- Influenza vaccine studies have poor quality and study conclusions often do not correspond with data in the study.

- Although 70% of studies had conclusions favorable to influenza vaccines, just 18% showed agreement between data reported and study conclusions. More than half of the studies were at high risk of bias.

- This paper found that higher quality influenza studies were a) significantly more likely to have conclusions corresponding to the data (OR = 16.35), and b) less likely to have conclusions supporting the vaccine's effectiveness.

- Influenza vaccine studies with favorable conclusions have significantly lower methodological quality.

- Influenza vaccine studies that receive funding by the industry are published in more prestigious journals with greater exposure and are cited more often than non-industry-sponsored studies of similar size and quality.

85.

Health authorities exaggerate the dangers of influenza and inflate the benefits of influenza vaccination

"The evidence that influenza represents a threat of public health proportions is questionable, the evidence that influenza vaccines reduce important patient-centered outcomes such as mortality is unreliable, the assumption that past influenza vaccine safety is predictive of future experience is unsound, and nonpharmaceutical interventions to manage influenza-like illness exist."

Doshi P. **Influenza vaccines: time for a rethink.** *JAMA Intern Med* 2013 Jun 10; 173(11): 1014-16.

- Influenza is less scary than advertised, influenza vaccines offer fewer benefits than expected, and the risks of vaccination should not be underestimated.
- Influenza vaccines provide no benefit to most recipients since a majority of people do not annually contract the disease.
- The "flu" (also known as influenza-like illness) has hundreds of causes. It should not be confused with influenza, which is just one of those causes.
- Influenza studies promoted by the CDC were shown to be substantially confounded by "healthy-user bias" (healthier people are more likely to get vaccinated), rendering the studies worthless.
- Influenza should not be called a "vaccine-preventable disease" since the vaccine is not very effective.
- Influenza vaccines can cause serious adverse effects and there is no reliable evidence that they can prevent dangerous complications of the disease.

86.

Marketing strategies designed to increase influenza vaccinations lack moral integrity and scientific support

"Closer inspection of influenza vaccine policies shows that although proponents employ the rhetoric of science, the studies underlying the policy are often of low quality and do not substantiate officials' claims. The vaccine might be less beneficial and less safe than has been claimed, and the threat of influenza appears overstated."

Doshi P. **Influenza: marketing vaccine by marketing disease.** *BMJ* 2013 May 16; 346: f 3037.

- In 1960, the CDC recommended influenza vaccinations for the elderly. By 2010, influenza vaccinations were urged for nearly everyone, including infants over the age of 6 months, children, teens, pregnant women (all trimesters), healthy adults, and healthcare workers.

- In 1990, 32 million doses of the influenza vaccine were available in the United States. By 2013, this number quadrupled to around 135 million doses, with vaccines administered in drug stores, supermarkets, and drive-throughs.

- The CDC claims that influenza vaccines can prevent up to 48% of deaths from all causes. However, non-CDC researchers realize that it's not possible for influenza vaccines to prevent nearly half of all deaths from all causes when influenza is estimated to only cause about 5% of all wintertime deaths.

- Thousands of people with influenza-like illness are tested every year. Only about 16% of all respiratory specimens test positive for influenza. The vaccine is not designed to protect against the other 84% of respiratory illnesses.

- There are no studies showing that influenza vaccines reduce serious outcomes in the elderly. The vaccine was approved for use based on its ability to induce antibodies, without evidence that those antibodies decrease illness.

- Influenza vaccines have been linked to febrile convulsions in young children and narcolepsy (a sleeping disorder) in adolescents.

87.

The CDC collaborates with vaccine manufacturers to increase uptake by intentionally using scare tactics and inflated influenza death figures

"U.S. data on influenza deaths are a mess. There are significant statistical incompatibilities between official estimates and national vital statistics data. Compounding these problems is a marketing of fear — a CDC communications strategy in which medical experts 'predict dire outcomes' during flu seasons."

Doshi P. **Are U.S. flu-death figures more PR than science?** *BMJ* 2005 Dec 10; 331: 1412.

- The CDC works on behalf of manufacturers by conducting well-coordinated scare campaigns to increase influenza vaccination.
- The CDC publicly asserts that influenza kills 36,000 Americans annually. However, the National Center for Health Statistics, operated by the CDC, shows an average of just 1,348 influenza deaths per year.
- CDC data on influenza are statistically biased, limiting the possibilities for rational discussion and reasonable public health policy.

Pertussis Mutations

Whole-cell pertussis vaccines (DTP) were introduced in the 1930s and 1940s to protect against whooping cough, a contagious disease that causes severe coughing attacks and labored breathing, conditions that can be deadly in infants. In the 1990s, a new acellular pertussis vaccine (DTaP) was introduced because some evidence revealed that it caused fewer adverse reactions. However, cases of whooping cough have increased throughout the world despite high vaccination rates against the disease.

Although health authorities often blame unvaccinated people for causing outbreaks of pertussis in vaccinated populations, studies in this chapter demonstrate that the pertussis vaccine was inadvertently designed to encourage evolutionary adaptation, which permitted virulent vaccine-resistant strains of pertussis to emerge. Other studies show that the vaccine increased cases of whooping cough caused by *B. parapertussis* — a cousin of *B. pertussis* — which the vaccine also is not effective against. Although cases of pertussis in unvaccinated children have increased, cases in vaccinated children have increased even more dramatically.

Perhaps the last two studies in this chapter are the most important. In the paper by Warfel and colleagues, baboons vaccinated against pertussis showed few symptoms of the disease but were highly infectious and spread pertussis to other baboons. In the paper by Althousse and Scarpino, epidemiological, genetic and mathematical data all converge to confirm asymptomatic transmission of pertussis from vaccinated individuals to other susceptible people. Both of these studies provide strong evidence that people who are vaccinated against pertussis may be silent carriers of the disease and capable of infecting others. They also suggest that herd immunity may not be possible with current acellular pertussis vaccines. Waning vaccine immunity, the evolutionary adaptation of *B. pertussis* to pertussis vaccinations, and the potential for vaccinated people to spread disease are important factors in the resurgence of whooping cough.

88.

Children who are fully vaccinated against pertussis are still susceptible to the disease

"Pertussis has increased in the U.S. since the 1980s despite high coverage with pertussis childhood vaccines. Protection from the DTaP series begins to wane after vaccination, contributing to the accumulation of vaccinated individuals who are still susceptible to disease."

Tartof SY, Lewis M, et al. **Waning immunity to pertussis following 5 doses of DTaP.** *Pediatrics* 2013 Apr; 131(4): e1047-52.

- This study assessed the risk in children of contracting pertussis within 6 years of receiving 5 recommended doses of the acellular pertussis vaccine (DTaP).
- In Minnesota children, the risk of pertussis doubled just two years after receiving the 5th dose of DTaP (risk ratio, RR = 1.9) and increased ninefold within six years after full vaccination (RR = 8.9). In Oregon children, the risk of pertussis quadrupled within six years after full vaccination (RR = 4.0).
- A resurgence of pertussis may be caused by several factors, including a true increase in disease, waning immunity, and changes in the pertussis organism — antigenic drift — away from targets of the vaccine.

89.

Acosta AM, DeBolt C, et al. **Tdap vaccine effectiveness in adolescents during the 2012 Washington state pertussis epidemic.** *Pediatrics* 2015 Jun; 135(6): 981-89.

"Tdap protection wanes within 2 to 4 years. Lack of long-term protection after vaccination is likely contributing to increases in pertussis among adolescents."

- This study investigated pertussis vaccine effectiveness in adolescents during a 2012 pertussis epidemic in Washington state.
- Within 2 to 4 years of receiving a sixth dose of an acellular pertussis vaccine (Tdap), vaccine effectiveness among adolescents declined to 34%.

90.

Outbreaks of pertussis are happening throughout the world despite high vaccination rates

"We show that global transmission of new [pertussis] strains is very rapid and that the worldwide population of B. pertussis is evolving in response to vaccine introduction. It seems plausible that the changes in the B. pertussis populations have reduced vaccine efficacy."

Bart MJ, Harris SR, et al. **Global population structure and evolution of *Bordetella pertussis* and their relationship with vaccination.** *MBio* 2014 Apr 22; 5(2): e01074.

- Outbreaks of whooping cough throughout the world are becoming increasingly more common, despite high vaccination rates.

- Researchers analyzed a worldwide collection of 343 strains of *B. pertussis* isolated between 1920 and 2010 to determine how the introduction of pertussis vaccines influenced adaptive behavior and the emergence of strains which produce more toxins.

- Antigenic divergence initially involved relatively few mutations but other newly predominant strains of pertussis toxins have emerged subsequent to pertussis vaccination.

- In many regions of the world, including Europe, the United States and Australia, new strains of pertussis have replaced common strains that were targeted by the pertussis vaccine.

- The evidence suggests that vaccination against whooping cough was the major factor inducing adaptive behavior in *B. pertussis* populations and a reduction in vaccine efficacy.

91.

A highly virulent strain of pertussis mutated from the pertussis vaccine and is causing new cases of the disease; the vaccine is not effective against the new strain

"Vaccines designed to reduce pathogen growth rate and/or toxicity may result in the evolution of pathogens with higher levels of virulence. We propose that waning immunity and pathogen adaptation have contributed to the resurgence of pertussis."

Mooi FR, van Loo IH, et al. ***Bordetella pertussis*** **strains with increased toxin production associated with pertussis resurgence.** *Emerg Infect Dis* 2009 Aug; 15(8): 1206-13.

- Several countries with highly vaccinated populations are experiencing a resurgence of pertussis.
- A highly virulent strain of pertussis toxin (ptxP3) recently emerged from within pertussis-vaccinated populations. (Due to pathogen adaptation, pertussis vaccination "may select for increased virulence.")
- The current pertussis vaccine offers some protection against the most common pertussis toxin (ptxP1) but not against the new, highly virulent strain.
- The new strain did not exist in the pre-vaccine era.
- The new strain produces 1.62 times more lethal toxin than the old strain.
- There is a statistically significant increase in hospitalizations and death caused by the new strain of pertussis when compared to the original strain.
- The new strain is responsible for increased cases of pertussis in all age groups.
- The replacement of ptxP1 by ptxP3 is now a global problem affecting at least four continents: Asia, Europe, North America and South America.

92.

Pertussis vaccines caused new, vaccine-resistant strains of pertussis to emerge, and increased cases of the disease

"Given that Bordetella pertussis has no non-human hosts or environmental niche, vaccine-mediated immunity is the most likely selective pressure against Bordetella pertussis."

Schmidtke AJ, Boney KO, et al. **Population diversity among *Bordetella pertussis* isolates, United States, 1935–2009**. *Emerg Infect Dis* 2012 August; 18(8): 1248-55.

- In the United States, the *Bordetella pertussis* population has evolved following the introduction of pertussis vaccines.
- The number of reported pertussis cases has increased since the early 1980s.
- Today, the commonly circulating strains of *Bordetella pertussis* vary from the strains that current pertussis vaccines were designed to fight against.
- The resurgence in cases of pertussis coincides with the emergence of virulent, non-vaccine strains of pertussis.
- *Bordetella pertussis* has no non-human host, so the selective pressures it confronts are limited to the human immune system and the pertussis vaccine.

93.

Mooi FR, Van Der Maas NA, De Melker HE. **Pertussis resurgence: waning immunity and pathogen adaptation — two sides of the same coin.** *Epidemiol Infect* 2014 Apr; 142(4): 685-94.

"Pertussis or whooping cough has persisted and resurged in the face of vaccination."

- After pertussis vaccines were introduced, antigenic divergence among vaccine strains of *Bordetella pertussis* occurred, and the production of pertussis toxin increased, significant factors in the persistence and resurgence of pertussis.

94.

Pertussis vaccine failures are due to genetic changes in pertussis strains and poor efficacy, not because too many people are unvaccinated

"Vaccine use has resulted in genetic changes in pertussis toxin, pertactin, and fimbriae [virulence factors] in circulating B. pertussis strains, and it has been suggested that this has led to increased vaccine failure rates."

Cherry JD. **Why do pertussis vaccines fail?** *Pediatrics* 2012 May 1; 129(5): 968-70. [Commentary.]

- Pertussis vaccines often fail to protect against whooping cough due to genetic changes in circulating strains of *Bordetella pertussis* and because *Bordetella parapertussis* now accounts for about 16.5% of coughing illnesses.

- Pertussis vaccines were not designed to protect against the new, genetically altered strains of *B. pertussis* nor against *B. parapertussis*.

- When the acellular pertussis vaccine (DTaP) replaced the whole cell pertussis vaccine (DTP) in the 1990s, the World Health Organization (WHO) created an official standard method to define cases of pertussis.

- The new case definition was excessively restrictive, requiring laboratory confirmation and at least 21 days of paroxysmal cough, eliminating legitimate cases of pertussis, artificially inflating the vaccine's reported efficacy.

- Pertussis vaccines also fail due to waning antibody levels over time.

- In a subset of one study, the true efficacy of the acellular pertussis vaccine was just 40%.

95.

Pertussis vaccines caused genetic changes in circulating strains of pertussis, which resulted in decreased vaccine efficacy (vaccine failures)

"We should consider the potential contribution of genetic changes in circulating strains of B. pertussis. It is clear that genetic changes have occurred over time in three B. pertussis antigens—pertussis toxin, pertactin, and fimbriae."

Cherry, JD. **Epidemic pertussis in 2012 — the resurgence of a vaccine-preventable disease**. *NEJM* 2012 Aug 30; 367(9): 785-87.

- Studies indicate that genetic changes in circulating strains of *B. pertussis* have led to vaccine failures.
- The number of *reported* pertussis cases and *actual* cases of *B. pertussis* infection should be considered separately.
- Only about 13% to 20% of prolonged cough illnesses in adolescents and adults are attributable to *B. pertussis* infection.

96.

Cherry JD. **Pertussis: challenges today and for the future.** *PLoS Pathog* 2013; 9(7): e1003418.

"The universal use of pertussis vaccines has been associated with genetic changes in circulating B. pertussis strains. Today with DTaP vaccines, genetic change should be a major concern regarding vaccine efficacy."

- Similar whooping cough illnesses can be caused by *Bordetella pertussis* and *Bordetella parapertussis*.
- Prior to major genetic changes in pertussis caused by the vaccine, efficacy was inflated by a stringent case definition established by WHO in 1991.

97.

Newly emerging, virulent strains of pertussis are resistant to the vaccine, reducing its effect on whooping cough

"The emergence of pertactin-deficient isolates in countries where the acellular vaccines were recently introduced is alarming."

Barkoff AM, Mertsola J, et al. **Appearance of *Bordetella pertussis* strains not expressing the vaccine antigen pertactin in Finland.** *Clin Vaccine Immunol* 2012 Oct; 19(10): 1703-04. [Correspondence.]

- Despite widespread pertussis vaccinations, a resurgence of whooping cough has been reported in several countries.
- In 2011, eight years after Finland introduced the acellular pertussis vaccine, non-pertactin-expressing *B. pertussis* strains were discovered.

98.

Queenan AM, Cassiday PK, Evangelista A. **Pertactin-negative variants of *Bordetella pertussis* in the United States.** *N Engl J Med* 2013 Feb 7; 368(6): 583-84. [Correspondence.]

"Although much attention has been given to the waning immunity associated with the introduction of acellular vaccines, another factor contributing to the outbreaks may be the adaptation of B. pertussis to vaccine selection pressure."

- Acellular pertussis vaccines are designed to protect against pertactin, a virulence factor of *B. pertussis*. However, vaccine-resistant pertactin-negative mutations have emerged in France, Japan, Finland, and the United States.
- Pertactin-negative mutations are infectious/transmissible in humans and lethal in mouse experiments.
- The next generation of pertussis vaccines will need to account for the rising prevalence and virulence of these new pertactin-negative strains.

99.

The pertussis vaccine is becoming less effective as it causes virulent new strains to emerge and prevail

"Human host factors (genetic factors and immune status) that select for pertactin-deficient strains have arisen. The most likely explanation for prevalence of pertactin-deficient strains is vaccine-driven selection."

Otsuka N, Han HJ, et al. **Prevalence and genetic characterization of pertactin-deficient *Bordetella pertussis* in Japan.** *PloS One* 2012; 7(2): e31985.

- Pertactin, a primary virulence factor of *B. pertussis*, causes whooping cough. In Japan and throughout the world, pertactin polymorphism (genetic variation) has significantly increased in *B. pertussis* populations following acellular pertussis vaccinations.
- Since the mid-1990s, the newly emerging non-vaccine type of pertactin (Prn2) has been replacing the vaccine-type of pertactin (Prn1).
- Scientists are concerned that the new pertactin-deficient strains can evade acellular pertussis vaccines, reducing their efficacy against whooping cough.

100.

Stefanelli P, Fazio C, et al. **A natural pertactin deficient strain of *Bordetella pertussis* shows improved entry in human monocyte-derived dendritic cells.** *New Microbiol* 2009 Apr; 32(2): 159-66.

"The results showed that this natural B. pertussis pertactin-deficient strain presented higher invasion ability. Five hours after infection, the pertactin-deficient strain had significantly increased invasion ability compared to the wild reference strain."

- This study compared the infective ability of a common *B. pertussis* strain of pertactin to a mutant "pertactin-deficient" strain of *B. pertussis*. The new strain can infect dendritic cells in humans with significantly more virulence than the common strain.

101.

Pertussis vaccines became less effective by causing strains of the disease to mutate, and shifted cases of whooping cough from children to older age groups

"Since the introduction of the acellular pertussis vaccines there has been a steady increase in the number of B. pertussis and B. parapertussis isolates collected that are lacking expression of pertactin. These isolates seem to be as virulent as those expressing all virulence factors according to animal and cellular models of infection."

Hegerle N, Paris AS, et al. **Evolution of French *Bordetella pertussis* and *Bordetella parapertussis* isolates: increase of Bordetellae not expressing pertactin**. *Clin Microbiol Infect* 2012 Sep; 18(9): E340-6.

- In France, whole-cell pertussis vaccination was initiated in 1959 and acellular pertussis vaccines were introduced in 1998. This paper analyzed changes in the adaptive behavior of bacterial agents that cause whooping cough.

- Whole-cell pertussis vaccination caused genetic mutations in the *B. pertussis* population. These genetic changes did not occur in areas where whole-cell pertussis vaccination rates were low.

- Since 2005, seven years after France started using acellular pertussis vaccines, new "pertactin-deficient" strains of *B. pertussis* and *B. parapertussis* emerged.

- Pertussis vaccine effectiveness is reduced by antigenic changes in *B. pertussis* and *B. parapertussis* strains.

- The French pertussis vaccination program decreased the incidence of pertussis among young children. However, during the next 20 years adolescents and adults became reservoirs for the disease and a threat to newborns.

- Pertussis vaccination programs in France created an obstacle that *Bordetella* populations had to surmount, promoting evolution and natural selection within these populations.

102.

Herd immunity may not be possible with vaccines that induce strains of pertussis to rapidly evolve and evade the vaccine

"This study and other studies have reported the increasing prevalence of isolates not expressing pertactin in many countries that have a high uptake of acellular pertussis vaccination. The overall effect of lack of expression of an antigen on herd immunity is unknown."

Lam C, Octavia S, et al. **Rapid increase in pertactin-deficient *Bordetella pertussis* isolates, Australia.** *Emerg Infect Dis* 2014 Apr; 20(4): 626-33.

- This study identified strains of pertussis collected in Australia from 1997 to 2012, after the acellular pertussis vaccine was introduced.

- From 2008 to 2012 there was a large outbreak of pertussis in Australia. Between 30% and 80% of all circulating pertussis strains were pertactin-deficient.

- Pertactin-deficient strains of pertussis have a high level of transmissibility, consistent with an increasing number of infections.

- Pertussis vaccine selection pressure, or vaccine-driven adaptation, induced the evolution of *B. pertussis,* the bacterium responsible for whooping cough.

103.

Octavia S, Sintchenko V, et al. **Newly emerging clones of *Bordetella pertussis* carrying prn2 and ptxP3 alleles implicated in Australian pertussis epidemic in 2008-2010.** *J Infect Dis* 2012 Apr 15; 205(8): 1220-24.

"Pertussis has reemerged as a significant public health threat in populations with historically high vaccine uptake. [New] isolates have the potential not only to evade the protective effects of the acellular pertussis vaccine but also to increase disease severity as a double act of B. pertussis adaptation."

104.

A resurgence of whooping cough is caused by waning vaccine immunity and small mutations in *B. pertussis* that evade pertussis vaccines

"Despite high vaccination coverage, pertussis has resurged and has become one of the most prevalent vaccine-preventable diseases in developed countries. We have proposed that both waning immunity and pathogen adaptation have contributed to the persistence and resurgence of pertussis."

van Gent M, Bart MJ, et al. **Small mutations in *Bordetella pertussis* are associated with selective sweeps.** *PloS One* 2012; 7(9): e46407.

- Despite high vaccination rates in The Netherlands and many other countries, cases of whooping cough are increasing.
- *Bordetella pertussis* (*B. pertussis*) is the main bacterial agent that causes whooping cough.
- This paper examined how more than 60 years of pertussis vaccination in The Netherlands has influenced the *B. pertussis* pathogen population.
- Between 1949 and 2010, *B. pertussis* in The Netherlands has consistently adapted to pertussis vaccinations and increased its fitness following several small mutations.
- Small mutations can induce significant alterations in bacterial pathogen populations within a time period of just 6 to 19 years.
- Waning vaccine immunity and the evolutionary adaptation of *B. pertussis* to pertussis vaccinations are important factors in the resurgence of whooping cough.

105.

DTaP vaccination to protect children from *B. pertussis* increases their risk of whooping cough from *B. parapertussis*

"There is evidence from both prospective epidemiological surveillance and recent experiments in model organisms that immunization with the acellular vaccine may actually increase the host's susceptibility to infection by B. parapertussis."

Lavine J, Broutin H, et al. **Imperfect vaccine-induced immunity and whooping cough transmission to infants.** *Vaccine* 2010 Dec 10; 29(1): 11-16.

- Cases of whooping cough have increased throughout the world despite high vaccination rates. This paper analyzed current and historical data on pertussis epidemiology to determine why pertussis vaccines are failing.
- Vaccine-induced immunity against pertussis is declining. The time between vaccination and infection — vaccine-failure — continues to shrink.
- It appears that vaccine-driven pathogen evolution selected for another species of pertussis — *B. parapertussis* — that can infect more efficiently.
- *B. parapertussis* mostly infects younger age groups that were repeatedly vaccinated against *B. pertussis*.
- The DTaP shot, designed to protect against *B. pertussis*, does not protect against whooping cough caused by *B. parapertussis*.
- In the pre-vaccine era, when *bordetella pertussis* freely circulated, people who contracted the disease remained immune from additional cases by getting natural immune boosts through frequent contact with infected people. Today, most people are vaccinated so natural boosts to immunity are rare.
- Infants are the only age group that has a significant risk of mortality from whooping cough.

106.

Pertussis vaccines do not protect against all strains of *B. pertussis* nor against *B. parapertussis*

"The antibody generated against B. pertussis proteins that offers protection against B. pertussis offers little protection against B. parapertussis infection. Our data indicate that B. parapertussis infections contribute significantly to the overall pertussis burden and contribute to the pool of children thought to have vaccine failure."

Cherry JD, Seaton BL. **Patterns of *Bordetella parapertussis* respiratory illnesses: 2008-2010.** *Clin Infect Dis* 2012 Feb 15; 54(4): 534-37.

- In the pre-vaccine era, nearly all cases of whooping cough were caused by *B. pertussis*. By 2010, 16.5% of cases were caused by *B. parapertussis*, for which vaccines offer little or no protection.
- About 95% of all *B. parapertussis* cases occur in children 10 years of age and younger.

107.

Guiso N. ***Bordetella pertussis* and pertussis vaccines.** *Clin Infect Dis* 2009 Nov 15; 49(10): 1565-69.

"The acellular pertussis-induced immune response targets the virulence of B. pertussis and not B. parapertussis, another causative agent of the disease. The possibility of B. parapertussis taking the place of B. pertussis must thus be considered."

- Acellular pertussis vaccines provide some protection against *B. pertussis* but not against *B. parapertussis,* which also causes whooping cough.
- Pertussis vaccines control some, *but not all,* strains that can cause whooping cough, enabling the bacterium to adapt and survive in humans.
- The strains of pertussis in circulation today are as virulent as the strains that were circulating during the pre-vaccine era.

108.

The acellular pertussis vaccine increased cases of whooping cough caused by *B. parapertussis*, which the vaccine is not effective against

"Following the increase of [acellular] pertussis vaccination coverage, we observed a relative increase of B. parapertussis cases in comparison to B. pertussis cases."

Liese JG, Renner C, et al. **Clinical and epidemiological picture of *B. pertussis* and *B. parapertussis* infections after introduction of acellular pertussis vaccines.** *Arch Dis Child* 2003 Aug; 88(8): 684-87.

- This study was designed to determine the clinical characteristics and relative frequency of *B. pertussis* and *B. parapertussis* disease in vaccinated and unvaccinated Germans after the introduction of acellular pertussis vaccines.
- Less than 5 years after widespread acellular pertussis vaccinations, whooping cough cases caused by *B. parapertussis* — rather than by *B. pertussis* — increased from 20% to 36%.
- About one-third of all children with *B. parapertussis* infection had typical whooping cough symptoms, including paroxysms, whooping, and vomiting.
- Sixty-two percent of all whooping cough cases caused by *B. pertussis* and 81% of all cases caused by *B. parapertussis* were fully vaccinated.
- The high rate of prior vaccination among the *B. parapertussis* cases indicates that the acellular pertussis vaccine has very low or no efficacy against whooping cough caused by *B. parapertussis*.
- Incomplete efficacy of the acellular pertussis vaccine is shifting *B. pertussis* infections to adolescents and adults.

109.

Acellular pertussis vaccination in mice increases susceptibility to whooping cough from *B. parapertussis* infection

"We conclude that acellular pertussis vaccination interferes with the optimal clearance of B. parapertussis and enhances the performance of this pathogen. Our data raise the possibility that widespread acellular pertussis vaccination can create hosts more susceptible to B. parapertussis infection."

Long GH, Karanikas AT, et al. **Acellular pertussis vaccination facilitates *Bordetella parapertussis* infection in a rodent model of bordetellosis.** *Proc Biol Sci* 2010 July 7; 277(1690): 2017-25.

- Acellular pertussis vaccines are designed to protect against whooping cough caused by *B. pertussis*. The vaccine does not protect against whooping cough caused by *B. parapertussis* and actually increases susceptibility to the disease.

- The purpose of this study was to determine how acellular pertussis vaccination increases host susceptibility to whooping cough from *B. parapertussis*.

- Two-hundred mice were divided into groups. Half the mice received 2 doses of an acellular pertussis vaccine; the other mice received a placebo. Three weeks later, some of the mice were infected with *B. pertussis*, others with *B. parapertussis*. The mice were then killed, their lungs removed and the number of invading bacteria counted.

- Results: vaccinated mice had a 40-fold increase in *B. parapertussis* bacterial colonization in their lungs compared to the unvaccinated mice.

- Acellular vaccination focuses immune responses on *B. pertussis,* impeding the immune system's ability to defend against *B. parapertussis*.

- Acellular pertussis vaccination shifts bacterial dominance from *B. pertussis* to *B. parapertussis,* raising the risk of treated people acquiring the infection.

- Future vaccination strategies must weigh the effects of natural selection.

110.

Pertussis vaccines do not protect against whooping cough caused by *B. holmesii*

"These findings indicate that B. holmesii is a widespread pathogen among populations that are highly vaccinated against B. pertussis."

Zhang X, Weyrich LS, et al. **Lack of cross-protection against *Bordetella holmesii* after pertussis vaccination.** *Emerg Infect Dis* 2012 Nov; 18(11): 1771-79.

- *Bordetella holmesii* is infecting humans in many parts of the world with whooping cough-like symptoms. However, the standard vaccine against *Bordetella pertussis* does not protect against this recently identified species.
- In this study, researchers gave mice acellular or whole-cell *B. pertussis* vaccines then exposed them to *B. holmesii*. Data indicate that *B. pertussis* vaccination is not protective against *B. holmesii* infections.

111.

Pittet LF, Emonet S, et al. ***Bordetella holmesii:* an under-recognised Bordetella species.** *Lancet Infect Dis* 2014 Jun; 14(6): 510-19.

"B. holmesii's adaptation to human beings is continuing, and virulence might increase."

- Some people misdiagnosed with *B. pertussis* are infected with *B. holmesii,* which may cause pertussis-like symptoms and invasive infections, such as bacteremia, pneumonia, meningitis, endocarditis, pericarditis, and arthritis. Pertussis-like infections due to *B. holmesii* may be underestimated.

112.

Kamiya H, Otsuka N, et al. **Transmission of *Bordetella holmesii* during pertussis outbreak, Japan.** *Emerg Infect Dis* 2012 Jul;18(7):1166-69.

"Epidemiologic links were found between 5 patients. B. holmesii may have been transmitted from person to person."

113.

Pertussis vaccines give imperfect immunity, which is causing outbreaks of whooping cough in highly vaccinated populations

"The fact that populations of B. pertussis may have evolved to circumvent the immune responses elicited by vaccination and to alter their virulence levels raises a number of questions concerning the design and use of future vaccines."

van Boven M, Mooi FR, et al. **Pathogen adaptation under imperfect vaccination: implications for pertussis.** *Proc Biol Sci* 2005 Aug 7; 272 (1572): 1617-24.

- Despite decades of pertussis vaccination, whooping cough is now a re-emerging problem in developed countries.

- This paper investigated the behavior of the *B. pertussis* pathogen population under pressure from vaccination.

- The acellular pertussis vaccine provides imperfect immunity, which is likely to increase pathogen circulation in vaccinated populations. Unvaccinated individuals in vaccinated populations are also at greater risk of infection.

- The *B. pertussis* strain of whooping cough appears to have evolved, altering virulence and evading vaccine protection.

- Although cases of pertussis in unvaccinated children have increased since 1995, cases in vaccinated children have increased even more dramatically.

- Pertussis is mainly occurring in vaccinated children, adolescents and adults.

- Pertussis vaccination campaigns may ultimately fail if immunity conferred by the vaccine is temporary and the transmission rate of pertussis infections in vaccinated populations is greater than in unvaccinated populations. Both of these conditions appear to be true.

114.

Baboons vaccinated against pertussis became carriers and spread the disease

"Our results suggest that in addition to the potential contribution of reduced efficacy and waning immunity of the acellular pertussis vaccine, its inability to prevent colonization and transmission provides a plausible explanation for pertussis resurgence."

Warfel JM, Zimmerman LI, et al. **Acellular pertussis vaccines protect against disease but fail to prevent infection and transmission in a non-human primate model.** *Proc Natl Acad Sci* 2014 Jan 14; 111(2): 787-92.

- Pertussis circulation remains high in countries with high vaccination rates.
- In this study, infant baboons were vaccinated against pertussis at 2, 4, and 6 months of age, then exposed to the disease one month later. They were not protected from *B. pertussis* colonization and asymptomatic infection.
- Twenty-four hours after the vaccinated baboons were exposed to pertussis and placed in cages, unvaccinated baboons were added to each cage. The vaccinated baboons infected them with the disease.
- Acellular pertussis-vaccinated baboons had high levels of bacteria in their respiratory systems and were contagious for several weeks after they were infected — even when they did not exhibit overt symptoms of the disease.
- The acellular pertussis vaccine induces an immune response inferior to natural infection. It is unable to prevent infection and transmission of pertussis.
- Antibody levels induced by vaccination do not correlate with protection.
- This study provides evidence that people vaccinated against pertussis may be asymptomatic carriers and contribute significantly to spreading the disease.
- This study provides evidence that a) herd immunity is not possible with current acellular pertussis vaccines, and b) cocooning — vaccinating people who have contact with infants — is unlikely to benefit infants, especially if vaccinated people who don't show symptoms can still spread the disease.

115.

People who are vaccinated against pertussis can still spread the disease, making herd immunity and eradication unattainable

"We conclude that asymptomatic transmission from acellular pertussis-vaccinated individuals to fully susceptible individuals provides the most parsimonious explanation for the observed resurgence of B. pertussis in the US and UK, the changes in age-specific attack rates, the observed increase in B. pertussis genetic variation, and the multiply demonstrated failure of cocooning unvaccinated infants."

Althouse BM, Scarpino SV. **Asymptomatic transmission and the resurgence of *Bordetella pertussis*.** *BMC Med* 2015 Jun 24; 13(1): 146.

- There has been an increase in the incidence of whooping cough. Three reasons are usually given to explain the rise in cases: 1) waning immunity following vaccination, 2) evolution of *B. pertussis,* and 3) low vaccination rates.

- The authors of this study provide evidence of a fourth reason to explain the resurgence of whooping cough: asymptomatic or subclinical transmission of *Bordetella pertussis*. Vaccinated individuals who don't exhibit signs of the disease are able to infect other people.

- Authors of this paper examined epidemiological and genetic data on pertussis, then constructed mathematical models of *B. pertussis* transmission to understand the public health consequences of asymptomatic spread of the disease.

- As acellular pertussis vaccination rates rise, asymptomatic infections increase nearly 30-fold.

- The documented failure of cocooning — vaccinating family members to protect newborns and infants — is compelling evidence for asymptomatic transmission of the disease from vaccinated individuals to susceptible people.

- This study provides a scientific explanation for *B. pertussis* genetic patterns, the failure of postnatal cocooning, the resurgence of whooping cough, and why herd immunity and eradication of the disease may be unattainable.

Pathogen Evolution and Imperfect Vaccines

An ideal vaccine would provide perfect protection that lasts for an entire lifetime. However, all vaccines are imperfect. They confer incomplete immunity. For example, some vaccines are designed to reduce — but not eliminate — the chances of becoming infected. Studies confirm that vaccines designed to reduce the growth rate of pathogens within their hosts produce conditions that actually increase pathogen virulence and prevent eradication of the disease.

Disease-causing organisms strive to maximally infect their hosts without killing them. They evolve to reduce virulence in non-immune (non-vaccinated or susceptible) populations and increase virulence when the host population is vaccinated or gains resistance. Thus, imperfect vaccines have non-intuitive consequences. They induce the targeted pathogen to adapt and evolve in unintended ways, creating undesirable disease outcomes in individuals and entire host populations.

The studies in this chapter provide strong evidence that imperfect vaccines promote the evolution of virulent pathogen strains that result in more severe and deadly infections. Herd immunity may never be achieved because high vaccination rates impel the pathogen family to avoid extinction by enhancing its hostile nature as it adapts to its new environment. If a true herd immunity threshold level is achieved, it will create a strong selective pressure that fosters the emergence of mutant strains. This adaptive behavior is favorable to the pathogen family but detrimental to vaccination campaign goals, affecting the overall or long-term burden of disease within both vaccinated and unvaccinated people.

116.

Imperfect vaccines promote the evolution of more virulent strains of the disease

"We explore the potential consequences of the use of imperfect vaccines. The use of these vaccines may drive the evolution of parasite virulence."

Gandon S, Mackinnon MJ, et al. **Imperfect vaccination: some epidemiological and evolutionary consequences.** *Proc Biol Sci* 2003 Jun 7; 270 (1520): 1129-36.

- Vaccines can be formulated to a) reduce the probability of becoming infected by a disease-causing pathogen, or b) diminish the growth rate of the pathogen residing within the human host.

- Different vaccination strategies have non-intuitive consequences for the evolution — adaptation — of the pathogen and the effects that vaccination will have on the *total* or *long-term* disease burden.

- Vaccines that are designed to reduce the growth rate of parasites within their hosts produce conditions that actually increase parasite virulence and prevent eradication of the disease.

- High vaccination rates, especially, can have negative consequences for the host population by enhancing the hostile nature of the parasite which can increase prevalence of the disease, precluding its elimination.

- Evolution impels the parasite family to avoid extinction by adapting to a new environment, the vaccinated hosts.

- Even when parasite evolution does not occur, intermediate vaccination rates in a host population may still cause negative consequences if the risk of serious illness increases with the age of the host.

117.

Vaccines that provide incomplete immunity encourage the evolution of more virulent pathogen strains and deadly infections

"Vaccines designed to reduce pathogen growth-rate and/or toxicity diminish selection against virulent pathogens. The subsequent evolution leads to higher levels of intrinsic virulence and hence to more severe disease in unvaccinated individuals. This evolution can erode any population-wide benefits such that overall mortality rates are unaffected, or even increase, with the level of vaccination coverage."

Gandon S, Mackinnon MJ, et al. **Imperfect vaccines and the evolution of pathogen virulence.** *Nature* 2001 Dec 13; 414(6865): 751-56.

- This paper studied imperfect vaccines and their potential to enhance the evolution of pathogen virulence increasing host mortality rates.
- Vaccines that do not provide full immunity must be reevaluated in light of these findings.

118.

Ganusov VV, Antia R. **Imperfect vaccines and the evolution of pathogens causing acute infections in vertebrates.** *Evolution* 2006 May; 60(5): 957-69.

"We find that the use of either anti-growth or anti-transmission vaccines leads to the evolution of pathogens with an increased within-host growth rate; infection of unvaccinated hosts with such evolved pathogens results in high host mortality."

- This paper analyzed vaccines that do not provide complete immunity to determine whether they encourage the evolution of more or less virulent pathogen strains.
- Imperfect vaccines promote the evolution of virulent pathogen strains that result in deadly infections.

119.

Population-wide vaccine-derived immunity promotes the evolution of novel and more virulent pathogen strains

"We experimentally tested whether immune pressure promotes the evolution of more virulent pathogens by evolving parasite lines in immunized and non-immunized ('naive') mice. We found that parasite lines evolved in immunized mice became more virulent to both naive and immune mice than lines evolved in naive mice."

Mackinnon MJ, Read AF. **Immunity promotes virulence evolution in a malaria model.** *PLoS Biol* 2004; 2(9): e230.

- Pathogens strive to maximally infect their hosts without killing them. They evolve to reduce virulence in susceptible (non-immune) populations and increase virulence when the host population is vaccinated or gains resistance.
- Pathogens in host populations with high immunity evolve more virulent strains than pathogens residing in naive or low immunity host populations.
- Immunity from disease can stimulate natural selection by continually evolving more aggressive parasites that circumvent immune defenses. These novel strains could have a selective advantage only in vaccinated hosts.

120.

Mackinnon MJ, Read AF. **Virulence in malaria: an evolutionary viewpoint.** *Philos Trans R Soc Lond B Biol Sci* 2004 Jun 29; 359(1446): 965-86.

"One implication of this evolutionary view of virulence is that parasite populations are expected to evolve new levels of virulence in response to medical interventions such as vaccines and drugs."

- Anti-toxin and anti-growth-rate vaccines reduce the probability that the parasite will kill its host which, in turn, encourages the parasite population to evolve more virulent strains.
- Vaccine-induced virulent strains impact immune and non-immune people.

121.

Herd immunity may never be achieved because high vaccination rates encourage the evolution of more severe disease-causing organisms

"A partially effective immune response — enough to exert selective pressure but not effective enough to suppress escape viral mutants — is the most effective driving force of antigenic variation."

Rodpothong P, Auewarakul P. **Viral evolution and transmission effectiveness.** *World J Virol* 2012 Oct 12; 1(5): 131-34.

- In theory, if enough people are vaccinated, herd immunity will be achieved and chains of infection will be disrupted. In reality, a true herd immunity threshold may never be reached within normal heterogenous populations.
- If a true herd immunity threshold level is achieved, it will create a strong selective pressure that encourages the emergence of mutant viral strains.

122.

André JB, Gandon S. **Vaccination, within-host dynamics, and virulence evolution.** *Evolution* 2006 Jan; 60(1): 13-23.

"We show that vaccination may promote the evolution of faster replicating and, consequently, more virulent strains. We also show that intermediate vaccination coverage may lead to the coexistence of two different parasite strategies (a low-virulence strain adapted to naive hosts, and a high-virulence strain, more generalist, adapted to both naive and vaccinated hosts)."

- This paper examined how vaccinations may promote the evolution of more severe disease.
- Different vaccination strategies under varying epidemiological conditions significantly alter disease outcomes in individuals and entire host populations.

123.

Vaccines alter the environment in which parasites live, promoting the evolution of more virulent strains

"Evolutionary ecologists would not find it surprising that the large epidemiological perturbations caused by vaccination also result in considerable changes in the way that natural selection acts on parasite populations. Since there is often substantial genetic variation in antigenic reactivity among parasite strains, vaccination will select for those strains that are able to evade the vaccine-induced immunological response mounted by hosts."

Gandon S, Day T. **The evolutionary epidemiology of vaccination.** *J R Soc Interface* 2007 Oct 22; 4(16): 803-17.

- The host environment where parasites live is significantly altered by vaccines.
- Disease virulence evolves due to restrictions placed on disease-causing organisms. Vaccines that restrain the growth of parasites induce them to adapt to their new environment, becoming more fit and severe.
- After a vaccine program begins, most infections occur in the non-vaccinated population. Since this group has fewer susceptible hosts to infect — and the parasite doesn't want to kill its host — lower virulence is selected. In contrast, the vaccinated population has greater immunity so new infections in this group can only occur if more transmissible, virulent strains are selected.

124.

Magori K, Park AW. **The evolutionary consequences of alternative types of imperfect vaccines.** *J Math Biol* 2014 Mar; 68(4): 969-87.

"The emergence and spread of mutant pathogens that evade the effects of prophylactic interventions, including vaccines, threatens our ability to control infectious diseases globally."

- Imperfect vaccines selectively favor the emergence of mutant pathogen strains, confirming a link between epidemiological and evolutionary dynamics.

125.

Pathogens evolve to become more virulent in immune populations, diminishing the benefits of vaccination

"Host immunity can exacerbate selection for virulence. Therefore, vaccines that reduce pathogen replication may select for more virulent pathogens, eroding the benefits of vaccination and putting the unvaccinated at greater risk."

Mackinnon MJ, Gandon S, Read AF. **Virulence evolution in response to vaccination: the case of malaria.** *Vaccine* 2008 Jul 18;26 Suppl 3:C42-52.

- Pathogens may become more virulent in an abnormal host environment, which can occur following a population-wide vaccination program.

- In this paper, scientists infected groups of mice with parasite clones to quantify the relationship between transmissibility, persistence and virulence of infection.

- Pathogens with ideal fitness are those with an intermediate level of virulence.

- The benefits of higher transmissibility and persistence only occur if the host survives. Pathogens that are too virulent will kill their hosts, halting infectious transmission.

- The most evolutionarily successful pathogen maximizes the duration of infection and its capacity to infect new hosts while suppressing virulence just enough to keep its host alive.

- In vaccinated populations where hosts are immune, pathogen variants with greater virulence can evolve because host death is less likely. In unvaccinated populations, host death is more likely, therefore virulent strains are restrained from emerging.

- The evolutionary consequences associated with the widespread use of vaccines where pathogens can be transmitted through vaccinated hosts need to be carefully weighed.

126.

Imperfect vaccines may cause a resurgence of disease

"The control of some childhood diseases has proved to be difficult even in countries that maintain high vaccination coverage. This may be due to the use of imperfect vaccines."

Magpantay FMG, Riolo MA, et al. **Epidemiological consequences of imperfect vaccines for immunizing infections.** *Siam J Appl Math* 2014; 74(6): 1810-30.

- No vaccine provides perfect protection that lasts for an entire lifetime. They all fail in some way.

- This paper systematically analyzed three different types of imperfect vaccines — leaky, all-or-nothing, and waning — to assess their different modes of failure, affect on herd immunity, and control of disease at the population level.

- Imperfect vaccines may a) reduce the probability of infection upon exposure, b) confer no protection to a percentage of vaccinated people, or c) provide protection that eventually wanes.

- Mathematical simulations indicate that some imperfect vaccines have a "honeymoon" time frame, a temporary period of low disease incidence following the initiation of vaccination campaigns.

- Honeymoon periods are followed by different modes of vaccine failure — failure in degree, in take, or duration — leading to a resurgence of disease at the population level, years or decades later.

Strain Replacement
Haemophilus influenzae

Vaccines that target some but not all strains of a disease can induce the emergence of other strains that become more prominent as they replace previous ones. Often, the new strains are more virulent and may infect age groups normally unaffected by the disease. This occurred following vaccination programs against *Haemophilus influenzae* type b (Hib) and pneumococcal disease.

Haemophilus influenzae (no relation to influenza) is a serious bacterial disease that can cause middle ear infections, respiratory infections, inflammation of the throat, and meningitis. There are several different strains of *Haemophilus influenzae*, including types a, b, c, d, e, f, and other non-typeable strains. In 1991, a vaccine targeting Hib was recommended for U.S. infants because this strain was the most common cause of bacterial meningitis. (The other strains rarely caused invasive disease.) Shortly thereafter, the Hib vaccine was introduced in many other countries around the world.

The studies in this section provide evidence that mass vaccinations against *Haemophilus influenzae* type b decreased cases of *Haemophilus influenzae* caused by the "b" strain (Hib) but increased deadly infections caused by the "a" strain (Hia) and other non-b strains. After years of vaccination against Hib, the emergence of *Haemophilus influenzae* due to non-b strains is causing global alarm. Invasive non-b strains of *Haemophilus influenzae* are more virulent, causing severe disease in the pediatric population. Adults and the elderly have also become more susceptible to invasive *Haemophilus influenzae* disease following Hib vaccinations of children. Strains infecting the elderly are especially severe, causing a significant increase in hospitalizations and death.

127.

Mass vaccination programs against *Haemophilus influenzae* type b (Hib) caused an increase in deadly infections from *Haemophilus influenzae* type a (Hia)

"Since introduction of the Haemophilus influenzae type b (Hib) conjugate vaccine, Haemophilus influenzae type a (Hia) infection has become a major invasive bacterial disease...."

Bruce MG, Zulz T, et al. ***Haemophilus influenzae* serotype a invasive disease, Alaska, USA, 1983-2011.** *Emerg Infect Dis* 2013; 19(6): 932-37.

- *Haemophilus influenzae* type a (Hia) infection mainly occurs in children under 2 years of age and is a serious disease, causing meningitis, hospitalization and death.
- In Alaska, 84% of the children infected with *Haemophilus influenzae* type a (Hia) were hospitalized, and the case-fatality rate was 9%.

128.

Ribeiro GS, Reis JN, et al. **Prevention of *Haemophilus influenzae* type b (Hib) meningitis and emergence of serotype replacement with type a strains after introduction of Hib immunization in Brazil.** *J Infect Dis* 2003 Jan 1; 187(1): 109-16.

"Haemophilus influenzae type b immunization contributed to an increased risk for Haemophilus influenzae type a meningitis."

- Mass vaccinations against *Haemophilus influenzae* type b decreased cases of *Haemophilus influenzae* caused by the "b" strain (Hib) while increasing cases caused by the "a" strain (Hia).
- The incidence of *Haemophilus influenzae* type a (Hia) meningitis increased 8-fold within one year after a vaccination program against *Haemophilus influenzae* type b (Hib) was initiated.

129.

Hib vaccination decreased cases of *Haemophilus influenzae* caused by the "b" strain but increased cases by other strains

"Vaccination against Hib has altered the epidemiology of invasive Haemophilus influenzae infections."

Adam HJ, Richardson SE, et al. **Changing epidemiology of invasive *Haemophilus influenzae* in Ontario, Canada: evidence for herd effects and strain replacement due to Hib vaccination.** *Vaccine* 2010 May 28; 28(24): 4073-78.

- *Haemophilus influenzae* type b vaccination reduced cases of Hib but increased cases of *Haemophilus influenzae* caused by non-typeable and "f" strains.
- Prior to infant vaccination against Hib, 65% of all *Haemophilus influenzae* cases were caused by the "b" strain. After Hib vaccination, 84% of all cases are now caused by the "f" strain and other non-b strains.

130.

Sadeghi-Aval P, Tsang RS, et al. **Emergence of non-serotype b encapsulated *Haemophilus influenzae* as a cause of pediatric meningitis in northwestern Ontario.** *Can J Infect Dis Med Microbiol* 2013 Spring; 24(1): 13-16.

"Before the introduction of the conjugate Hib vaccines, Hib was the leading cause of invasive bacterial disease in children younger than five years of age. In the post-Hib vaccine era, non-serotype b strains have become the primary cause of invasive Haemophilus influenzae disease. The shift toward more virulent non-serotype b strains may be a result of capsule switching or replacement."

- Following years of vaccination against Hib, the emergence of *Haemophilus influenzae* due to non-b strains is causing global alarm.
- Invasive non-b strains of *Haemophilus influenzae* are more virulent, causing severe disease in the pediatric population.

131.

Hib vaccinaton programs for children increased cases of invasive *Haemophilus influenzae* infections in adults

"Though numbers of Haemophilus influenzae type b (Hib) infections in adults fell after the introduction of Hib vaccines for children...total numbers of invasive Haemophilus influenzae infections increased due to a large rise in infections caused by non-capsulated Haemophilus influenzae strains."

Sarangi J, Cartwright K, et al. **Invasive *Haemophilus influenzae* disease in adults.** *Epidemiol Infect* 2000 Jun; 124(3): 441-47.

- After a national program to vaccinate children against *Haemophilus influenzae* type b (Hib) was introduced, the overall number of invasive *Haemophilus influenzae* infections in adults increased.

132.

Rubach MP, Bender JM, et al. **Increasing incidence of invasive *Haemophilus influenzae* disease in adults, Utah, USA.** *Emerg Infect Dis* Sep 2011; 17(9): 1645-50.

"As the prevalence of Hib has decreased [through vaccination], other encapsulated serotypes seem to have emerged as major causes of invasive disease, including Hif in Illinois and Hia in Brazil, Manitoba, and Northwestern Ontario."

- Adults have become more susceptible to invasive *Haemophilus influenzae* disease following Hib vaccinations of children.

- Most *Haemophilus influenzae* cases are now caused by increases in non-b strains, occur in the elderly population, and have high mortality.

- The increased cases of virulent non-type b *Haemophilus influenzae* among adults could be caused by the loss of cross-immunity that was provided by natural exposure to Hib or from changes in the organisms.

133.

Hib vaccines given to children caused increased cases of severe non-Hib infections in other age groups

"The clinical burden of invasive non-type b Haemophilus influenzae disease, measured as days of hospitalization/100,000 individuals at risk and year, increased significantly throughout the study period."

Resman F, Ristovski M, et al. **Invasive disease caused by *Haemophilus influenzae* in Sweden 1997-2009; evidence of increasing incidence and clinical burden of non-type b strains.** *Clin Microbiol Infect* 2011 Nov; 17(11): 1638-45.

- After vaccinating children against *Haemophilus influenzae* type b (Hib), researchers discovered a statistically significant increase in cases of invasive *Haemophilus influenzae* disease in the elderly, caused by *Haemophilus influenzae* type f (Hif) and non-typeable strains.

- The new strains are severe. More than one-third of the Hif cases and one-fifth of the non-typeable cases required intensive care.

134.

Shuel M, Hoang L, et al. **Invasive *Haemophilus influenzae* in British Columbia: non-Hib and non-typeable strains causing disease in children and adults.** *Int J Infect Dis* 2011 Mar; 15(3): e167-73.

"Invasive Haemophilus influenzae disease in a population vaccinated against Hib...involved both non-typeable and encapsulated strains. Adults were susceptible to invasive diseases due to non-typeable and serotype b and f strains, while in children, most diseases were due to serotype a bacteria."

- Following Hib vaccinations in children, there was an increase in non-Hib and non-typeable cases of *Haemophilus influenzae* in children and adults.

- Non-typeable strains of *Haemophilus influenzae* are resistant to antibiotics.

135.

Hib vaccines for children caused more fatal cases of non-Hib infections in the elderly

"The epidemiological characteristics of invasive H. influenzae disease have changed from a disease that predominantly affects children and is dominated by type b to a disease that predominantly affects adults and is dominated by non-typeable strains."

Dworkin MS, Park L, Borchardt SM. **The changing epidemiology of invasive *Haemophilus influenzae* disease, especially in persons > or = 65 years old.** *Clin Infect Dis* 2007 Mar 15; 44(6): 810-16.

- Following Hib vaccinations in children, cases of *Haemophilus influenzae* that were caused by non-type b (types a, c, d, e, f and non-typeable strains) significantly increased in adults and the elderly.

- The elderly were nearly 4 times more likely to get *Haemophilus influenzae* in 2004 than 9 years earlier (OR = 3.6). The case-fatality rate was 21%.

136.

Zanella RC, Bokermann S, et al. **Changes in serotype distribution of *Haemophilus influenzae* meningitis isolates identified through laboratory-based surveillance following routine childhood vaccination against *H. influenzae* type b in Brazil.** *Vaccine* 2011 Nov 8; 29(48): 8937-42.

"Following routine childhood vaccination against Haemophilus influenzae type b (Hib) disease...passive laboratory surveillance reported increasing numbers of non-b serotypes and non-typeable Haemophilus influenzae from meningitis cases."

- Prior to vaccination against Hib, 98% of all cases of *Haemophilus influenzae* meningitis were caused by the b strain. After vaccination, non-b and non-typeable serotypes accounted for 41% of all cases.

- The incidence of non-typeable *Haemophilus influenzae* meningitis increased in several age groups.

Strain Replacement
Pneumococcal disease

Pneumococcal disease, or *Streptococcus pneumoniae,* is a serious bacterial illness that can cause ear infections, blood infections, pneumonia, and meningitis. The pneumococcal pathogen consists of approximately 90 different strains. In 2000, a vaccine that targeted seven of these strains (PCV7) was licensed and recommended for U.S. infants. However, strains of *Streptococcus pneumoniae* are in strong competition with each other, which explains why non-vaccine strains rapidly replaced strains targeted by the vaccine. Thus, in 2010 a new vaccine that targeted 13 pneumococcal strains (PCV13) was introduced in the United States, United Kingdom and Canada. Today, pneumococcal vaccines are utilized by many countries around the world.

The studies in this section provide evidence that the pneumococcal vaccine reduced cases of pneumococcal disease caused by some strains but increased cases caused by others. Pneumococcal disease rates initially declined following universal vaccination of children against the disease but increased when non-vaccine strains quickly replaced strains targeted by the vaccine, rendering the vaccine inadequate. Some of the new strains that emerged are highly virulent and resistant to antibiotics. Pneumococcal vaccination of children also significantly increased the risk of invasive pneumococcal disease in adults. Vaccine-induced, life-threatening pneumococcal strains are now a worldwide problem.

137.

The pneumococcal vaccine (PCV7) reduced cases of pneumococcal disease caused by some strains but increased cases caused by other strains

"The introduction of a hepatavalent pneumococcal conjugate vaccine (PCV7) in 2000 in the USA has had a significant impact on decreasing the incidence of serious and invasive pneumococcal disease in all age groups, especially in children under 2 years of age. However, the emergence of replacement non-vaccine pneumococcal serotypes (e.g., 19A, 3, 15 and 33) has resulted in an increase in the incidence of serious and invasive infections."

Tan TQ. **Serious and invasive pediatric pneumococcal disease: epidemiology and vaccine impact in the USA.** *Expert Rev Anti Infect Ther* 2010 Feb; 8(2): 117-25.

- Despite years of vaccination against *Streptococcus pneumoniae,* serious and invasive pneumococcal infections continue to cause morbidity and mortality throughout the world.

138.

Mehtälä J, Antonio M, et al. **Competition between *Streptococcus pneumoniae* strains: implications for vaccine-induced replacement in colonization and disease.** *Epidemiology* 2013 Jul; 24(4): 522-29.

Vaccine-induced replacement by non-vaccine serotypes in pneumococcal colonization and disease poses a threat to the long-term effectiveness of pneumococcal vaccination."

- Strains of *Streptococcus pneumoniae* (pneumococcal disease) are in strong competition with each other, which explains why non-vaccine strains rapidly replace strains targeted by the pneumococcal vaccine.

139.

The pneumococcal vaccine (PCV7) reduced cases of invasive pneumococcal disease in children but significantly increased cases in adults

"Gains in disease reduction [following universal pneumococcal vaccination] were offset by increases in replacement serotypes, particularly among the over-65 age group."

Sahni V, Naus M, et al. **The epidemiology of invasive pneumococcal disease in British Columbia following implementation of an infant immunization program: increases in herd immunity and replacement disease.** *Can J Public Health* 2012 Jan-Feb; 103(1): 29-33.

- Shortly after a mass vaccination program targeting pneumococcal disease was initiated in British Columbia, the vaccine induced serotype replacement.
- Strains of *Streptococcus pneumoniae* that were not targeted by the vaccine replaced strains that were targeted, causing new cases of pneumococcal disease in elderly persons.

140.

Norton NB, Stanek RJ, et al. **Routine pneumococcal vaccination of children provokes new patterns of serotypes causing invasive pneumococcal disease in adults and children.** *Am J Med Sci* 2013 Feb; 345(2): 112-20.

"By 6 to 10 years after the initiation of pneumococcal vaccination, invasive pneumococcal disease (IPD) in children decreased significantly, whereas IPD in adults increased significantly."

- Infant vaccinations against *Streptococcus pneumoniae* induced a major shift in the prevalent strains responsible for causing pneumococcal disease.
- Adults are especially at risk of invasive pneumococcal disease caused by vaccine-induced replacement serotypes.

141.

The pneumococcal vaccine (PCV7) caused highly virulent, antibiotic resistant strains of pneumococcal disease to emerge

"This study shows rapid, nearly complete replacement of colonizing pneumococcal conjugate vaccine (PCV7) strains by non-PCV7 strains in young children. Some previously common risk factors for carriage have changed, which suggests that serotype changes may be challenging our previous knowledge of pneumococcal transmission."

Huang SS, Hinrichsen VL, et al. **Continued impact of pneumococcal conjugate vaccine on carriage in young children.** *Pediatrics* 2009 Jul; 124(1): e1-11.

- Invasive pneumococcal disease rates initially declined following universal vaccination of children against the disease but increased when non-vaccine strains quickly replaced strains targeted by the vaccine.
- There is evidence that antibiotic-resistant strains of invasive pneumococcal disease have arisen from recombinations of vaccine and non-vaccine strains.

142.

Dagan R. **Serotype replacement in perspective.** *Vaccine* 2009 Aug 21; 27 Suppl 3: C22-24.

"An increase in the incidence of invasive pneumococcal disease caused by non-vaccine serotypes — serotype replacement — has been observed since the introduction of the 7-valent pneumococcal conjugate vaccine (PCV7)."

- The non-vaccine strains are targeting children with underlying medical conditions and the elderly.
- Strain 19A, which is increasingly resistant to antibiotics, is a growing threat to both vaccinated and unvaccinated populations.

143.

Strain replacement from pneumococcal vaccination is a worldwide problem

"Our data identified an unexpected pattern of pneumococcal serotype replacement following PCV7. Continuous monitoring of pneumococcal carriage is important for decisions regarding the future of national vaccination policy in Japan."

Oikawa J, Ishiwada N, et al. **Changes in nasopharyngeal carriage of *Streptococcus pneumoniae*...in Japan.** *J Infect Chemother* 2014 Feb; 20(2): 146-49.

- The 7 strains of pneumococcus targeted by the vaccine virtually disappeared, but the overall pneumococcal rate did not change due to strain replacement.

144.

Alexandre C, Dubos F, et al. **Rebound in the incidence of pneumococcal meningitis in northern France: effect of serotype replacement.** *Acta Paediatr* 2010 Nov; 99(11): 1686-90.

"The incidence of pneumococcal meningitis in infants has rebounded in northern France during the pneumococcal conjugate vaccine program, with the emergence of non-vaccine pneumococcal serotypes."

145.

Melegaro A, Choi YH, et al. **Dynamic models of pneumococcal carriage and the impact of the heptavalent pneumococcal conjugate vaccine on invasive pneumococcal disease.** *BMC Infect Dis* 2010 Apr 8; 10: 90.

"This analysis suggests that a pneumococcal conjugate vaccination program would eradicate vaccine serotypes from circulation. However, the increase in carriage of non-vaccine serotypes, and the consequent increase in invasive disease, could reduce, negate or outweigh the benefit."

146.

PCV13 displaced PCV7 due to rapid strain replacement but is not expected to have much effect on reducing the overall burden of pneumococcal disease

"Introduction of the 13-valent pneumococcal conjugate vaccine (PCV13) did not affect the rate of overall pneumococcal colonization."

Lee GM, Kleinman K, et al. **Impact of 13-valent pneumococcal conjugate vaccination on *Streptococcus pneumoniae* carriage in young children in Massachusetts.** *J Pediatric Infect Dis Soc* 2014 Mar; 3(1): 23-32.

- In April 2010, a pneumococcal vaccine (PCV13) targeting 13 strains replaced the previous pneumococcal vaccine (PCV7) that targeted just 7 strains.
- Pneumococcal strains targeted by PCV13 were reduced in healthy children 6-23 months old but non-vaccine strains increased for all children.
- The vaccine had no efficacy in older children and some of the non-vaccine strains are resistant to antibiotics.

147.

Bottomley C, Roca A, et al. **A mathematical model of serotype replacement in pneumococcal carriage following vaccination.** *J R Soc Interface* 2013 Oct 16; 10(89): 20130786.

"The pneumococcal conjugate vaccines that are currently in use only protect against some serotypes of the bacterium, and there is now strong evidence that those serotypes not included in the vaccine increase in prevalence among most vaccinated populations."

- Evidence suggests that universal vaccination with PCV13 — the vaccine that targets 13 strains of *Streptococcus pneumoniae* — will barely reduce the overall prevalence of pneumococcal disease because the decrease in vaccine-targeted strains will be counteracted by an increase in non-vaccine strains.

148.

PCV13, like PCV7, is expected to continue inducing rapid strain replacement, rendering the new vaccine inadequate against pneumococcal disease

"As PCV13 use increases during the next several years, we anticipate that overall rates of colonization may transiently drop, but eventual non-PCV13 serotype replacement may occur."

Wroe PC, Lee GM, et al. **Pneumococcal carriage and antibiotic resistance in young children before 13-valent conjugate vaccine.** *Pediatr Infect Dis J* 2012 March; 31(3): 249-54.

- Seven years after PCV7 was introduced, all strains targeted by the vaccine were rapidly and nearly completely replaced by non-targeted strains.
- Although PCV7 caused an initial decline in strains of pneumococcus targeted by the vaccine, the overall pneumococcus carriage rate quickly returned to pre-PCV7 levels due to replacement by non-vaccine strains.
- The non-vaccine strains that replaced the targeted vaccine strains are increasingly resistant to antibiotics.

149.

Ricketson LJ, Wood ML, et al. **Trends in asymptomatic nasopharyngeal colonization with *Streptococcus pneumoniae* after introduction of the 13-valent pneumococcal conjugate vaccine in Calgary, Canada.** *Pediatr Infect Dis J* 2014 Jul; 33(7): 724-30.

"Pneumococcal nasopharyngeal colonization has changed profoundly since the introduction of conjugate vaccines.... By 2012, non-vaccine serotypes have nearly completely replaced vaccine serotypes. The impact on clinical disease remains to be seen."

- Just two years after PCV13 was introduced, 94% of all pneumococcal strains in healthy children were non-vaccine targeted serotypes.

150.

Vaccines against pneumococcal disease — PCV7 and PCV13 — have created a worldwide arms race against serious and invasive pneumococcal strains

"Vaccination against few serotypes can lead to elimination of the vaccine types and induces replacement by others."

Flasche S, Edmunds WJ, et al. **The impact of specific and non-specific immunity on the ecology of *Streptococcus pneumoniae* and the implications for vaccination.** *Proc Biol Sci* 2013 Oct 2; 280(1771): 20131939.

- The pneumococcal pathogen family consists of more than 90 different strains.
- Strain replacement is inevitable when vaccines only target some of the many strains that are in competition with each other.
- Non-vaccine strains have replaced strains targeted by the first-generation pneumococcal vaccine (PCV7), so new vaccines (PCV10, 13, 15, etc.) against additional strains are now being deployed in nations across the world, causing a multi-strain arms race.

151.

Tan TQ. **Pediatric invasive pneumococcal disease in the United States in the era of pneumococcal conjugate vaccines.** *Clin Microbiol Rev* 2012 July; 25(3): 409-19.

"The licensure (in 2000) and subsequent widespread use of a heptavalent pneumococcal conjugate vaccine (PCV7) have had a significant impact on decreasing the incidence of serious invasive pneumococcal disease in all age groups, especially in children under 2 years of age. However, the emergence of replacement non-PCV7 serotypes, especially serotype 19A, has resulted in an increase in the incidence of serious and invasive infections."

- PCV13 is expected to induce strain replacement like that seen with PCV7.

Human Papillomavirus (HPV)

Human papillomavirus (HPV) is a sexually transmitted virus that is spread through genital contact, usually by sexual intercourse. There are more than 100 subtypes of HPV. Some forms of the virus can cause abnormal cell growth on the lining of the cervix — cervical dysplasia — that years later can turn into cancer. However, in most cases the infections are harmless and go away without treatment. The body's own defense system eliminates the virus. Often, women experience no signs, symptoms or health problems.

In 2006, the Food and Drug Administration (FDA) approved a new HPV vaccine for 9- to 26-year-old girls and women. It was designed to protect against four of the more than 100 different HPV strains. Another HPV vaccine, produced by a U.K. manufacturer, is also available in many parts of the world.

The evidence presented in this chapter shows that clinical trials and marketing tactics by the HPV vaccine manufacturer may not be reliable. The HPV vaccine has been linked to serious adverse events, including autoimmune disorders, multiple sclerosis (MS), amyotrophic lateral sclerosis (ALS), Guillain-Barré syndrome (GBS), paralysis, convulsions, chronic fatigue syndrome, anaphylaxis, pulmonary embolisms and death. Malfunctions of the autonomic nervous system, cognitive dysfunctions, gait disturbances, menstrual problems and ovarian failure have all been reported following HPV vaccination as well.

Young teenage girls have no risk of dying from cervical cancer but they gamble with permanently disabling autoimmune or degenerative disorders, or death, following their HPV vaccines. In fact, the HPV vaccine may enhance cervical disease in young women with pre-existing HPV infections. In addition, the vaccine is unlikely to significantly reduce already low cervical cancer rates in countries with routine Pap screening.

152.

Clinical trials show no evidence that HPV vaccination can prevent cervical cancer; serious adverse reactions are common

"Current worldwide HPV immunization practices with either of the two HPV vaccines appear to be neither justified by long-term health benefits nor economically viable, nor is there any evidence that HPV vaccination (even if proven effective against cervical cancer) would reduce the rate of cervical cancer beyond what Pap screening has already achieved."

Tomljenovic L, Shaw CA. **Human papillomavirus (HPV) vaccine policy and evidence-based medicine: are they at odds?** *Ann Med* 2013 Mar; 45(2): 182-93.

- There is no significant evidence showing that HPV vaccination can prevent cervical cancer. The long-term benefits of HPV vaccination are based on assumptions, not reliable research data.

- The HPV vaccine has been linked to serious adverse reactions, including multiple sclerosis, autoimmune disorders, ALS, paralysis, convulsions, GBS, chronic fatigue syndrome, anaphylaxis, pulmonary embolisms and death.

- The HPV vaccine may actually enhance cervical disease in young women with pre-existing HPV-16/18 infections yet the FDA does not require pre-screening for these infections prior to vaccination.

- In Western nations, cervical cancer is rare. Mortality rates from the disease are much lower than the rate of reported serious adverse reactions, including deaths, from HPV vaccination.

- Pap screening in developed nations contributed to a 70% decline in cervical cancer in the past 50 years. HPV vaccination is unlikely to significantly reduce already low cervical cancer rates in countries with routine Pap screening.

- Health officials have not shown that HPV vaccination is safe nor that it can prevent cervical cancer. A science-based rationale for HPV vaccination does not exist, and ethical guidelines for informed consent may have been violated.

153.

HPV vaccine studies are flawed, resulting in unreliable safety and efficacy data

"Contrary to assertions from the vaccine manufacturers, as well as strong recommendations from health agencies worldwide, currently there is no evidence that vaccination with either Gardasil or Cervarix would have any notable impact in reducing the cervical cancer burden, at least not in countries with regular screening programs."

Tomljenovic L, Spinosa JP, Shaw CA. **Human papillomavirus (HPV) vaccines as an option for preventing cervical malignancies: (how) effective and safe?** *Curr Pharm Des* 2013 Mar; 19(8): 1466-87.

- The proclaimed benefits of HPV vaccination are predicated on unproven assumptions and contradict factual evidence. HPV vaccine safety and efficacy studies were poorly designed and inadequate.
- The FDA licensed the HPV vaccine based on safety and efficacy studies that were designed, sponsored and conducted by the vaccine manufacturer.
- HPV vaccines were associated with more than 60% of all life-threatening adverse reactions (including death) reported after vaccines and 82% of all reported permanent disability in females under 30 years of age.
- The HPV vaccine has negative efficacy and may exacerbate cervical disease in females who were already exposed to HPV strains targeted by the vaccine.
- Young teenage girls have zero risk of dying from cervical cancer but gamble with permanently disabling autoimmune or degenerative disorders, or death, following their HPV vaccines.
- Clinical trials have not provided evidence that the HPV vaccine has prevented a single case of cervical cancer or cervical cancer death.
- Cervical cancer will not develop in most women even with high-risk HPVs.
- Pap screening is effective. About 90% of cervical cancer deaths occur in developing nations without routine Pap screening programs.

154.

The HPV vaccine may cause lupus and other serious autoimmune diseases

"The present study provides epidemiological evidence supporting a significant relationship between HPV4 vaccine administration and serious autoimmune adverse events."

Geier DA, Geier MR. **A case-control study of quadrivalent human papillomavirus vaccine-associated autoimmune adverse events.** *Clin Rheumatol* 2015 Jul; 34(7): 1225-31.

- Researchers conducted an epidemiological case-control study of the Vaccine Adverse Event Reporting System (VAERS) to determine whether the HPV vaccine can induce serious autoimmune adverse events. A total of 22,011 adverse event reports in females 18 to 39 years of age were analyzed.

- Women diagnosed with systemic lupus erythematosus, a serious autoimmune disease, were 5 times more likely than controls to have received the HPV vaccine (odds ratio, OR = 5.3).

- Women diagnosed with alopecia (OR = 8.3), gastroenteritis (OR = 4.6), vasculitis (OR = 4.0), and central nervous system conditions (OR = 1.8) were also significantly more likely than controls to have received the HPV vaccine.

- Women diagnosed with Guillain-Barré syndrome, thrombocytopenia, conjunctivitis or diarrhea were not more likely than controls to have received the HPV vaccine.

- Vasculitis, gastroenteritis, and systemic lupus erthyematosus were associated with the highest percentages of life threatening outcomes. Central nervous system conditions, vasculitis, and arthritis were associated with the highest percentages of permanent disabilities.

- The median onset of symptoms following HPV vaccination was 6 days for vasculitis, 19 days for lupus, and 55 days for arthritis.

- The findings in this study are consistent with the known biological plausibility of vaccines to induce serious autoimmune adverse events in some people.

155.

The HPV vaccine may cause autoimmune diseases such as lupus and fatal cerebral vasculitis

"Based on the current data, a causal link between HPV vaccination and onset or relapse of systemic lupus erythematosus is plausible."

Gatto M, Agmon-Levin N, et al. **Human papillomavirus vaccine and systemic lupus erythematosus.** *Clin Rheumatol* 2013 Sep; 32(9): 1301-7.

- In this paper, researchers investigated the medical histories of six women who developed autoimmune symptoms compatible with systemic lupus erythematosus (SLE) following HPV vaccination.
- Health practitioners need to realize that the onset or exacerbation of autoimmune disease can occur following HPV vaccination.
- Risk factors associated with post-vaccination autoimmunity, such as genetic susceptibility, need to be determined.

156.

Tomljenovic L, Shaw CA. **Death after quadrivalent human papillomavirus (HPV) vaccination: causal or coincidental?** *Pharmaceut Reg Affairs* 2012; S12: 001.

"Our study suggests that HPV vaccines containing HPV-16L1 antigens pose an inherent risk for triggering potentially fatal autoimmune vasculopathies."

- In this paper, researchers analyzed brain samples of two young women who died following HPV vaccination. An immunohistochemical analysis showed evidence of an autoimmune vasculitis potentially triggered by HPV-16L1 antibodies binding to the wall of cerebral blood vessels.
- HPV vaccination may induce fatal autoimmune and neurological events. Doctors should be aware of this association.

157.

The HPV vaccine may cause chronic pain, fatigue and nervous system damage

"Clinicians should be aware of the possible association between HPV vaccination and the development of difficult to diagnose painful dysautonomic syndromes."

Martínez-Lavín M. **Hypothesis: Human papillomavirus vaccination syndrome — small fiber neuropathy and dysautonomia could be its underlying pathogenesis.** *Clin Rheumatol* 2015 Jul; 34(7): 1165-69.

- Adverse reactions following HPV vaccination appear to be more common when compared to other vaccinations.
- Symptoms often reported after HPV vaccination include chronic pain with parethesia, headaches, fatigue, fibromyalgia, and orthostatic intolerance (dizziness, heart palpitations and cognitive impairment upon standing upright).
- These debilities are difficult to diagnose although they may be related to dysfunctions of the sympathetic nervous system.

158.

Brinth LS, Pors K, et al. **Orthostatic intolerance and postural tachycardia syndrome as suspected adverse effects of vaccination against human papilloma virus.** *Vaccine* 2015 May 21; 33(22): 2602-5.

- In this paper, researchers examined 35 female patients who had symptoms consistent with autonomic dysfunction following HPV vaccination, and they described their common symptoms.
- All of the patients had orthostatic intolerance. Other symptoms included chronic headache, fatigue, cognitive dysfunction, neuropathic pain, and postural orthostatic tachycardia syndrome (POTS).
- Most of the patients had a high level of physical activity prior to HPV vaccination.

159.

Damage to the autonomic nervous system has been consistently reported after HPV vaccination, causing muscle weakness, fatigue, pain, and menstrual problems

"We suggest that the pathogenic alteration [after HPV vaccination] is located in the autonomic nervous system."

Brinth L, Theibel AC, et al. **Suspected side effects to the quadrivalent human papilloma vaccine.** *Dan Med J* 2015 Apr; 62(4): A5064.

- After Denmark initiated an HPV vaccination program, a collection of symptoms indicative of a malfunctioning autonomic nervous system began to manifest in some recipients of the vaccine.

- In this paper, researchers examined 53 female patients with suspected neurological side effects to the HPV vaccine, and they described their common symptoms.

- Symptoms included headaches, orthostatic intolerance, syncope, fatigue, cognitive dysfunction, insomnia, sensitivity to light, abdominal pain, neuropathic pain, chest pain, tremors, twitches, muscle weakness, difficulty walking, irregular periods, dry mouth, and hyperventilation.

- All of the patients reported the onset of symptoms within two months after receiving an HPV vaccine. The mean time between vaccination and onset of symptoms was 11 days.

- There was a high degree of consistency in the symptoms experienced by the patients. Mass psychogenic illness is an unlikely explanation.

- Prior to the onset of symptoms, patients in this study had high levels of physical activity. After their symptoms occurred, 98% were unable to continue daily activities and 75% had to quit school or work for at least 2 months.

- Patients with known chronic diseases prior to vaccination were excluded from analysis.

160.

The HPV vaccine may cause nerve damage, limb pain, menstrual problems, chronic fatigue and other adverse reactions

"A relatively high incidence of chronic limb pain, frequently complicated by violent, tremulous involuntary movements, has been noted in Japanese girls following HPV vaccination."

Kinoshita T, Abe RT, et al. **Peripheral sympathetic nerve dysfunction in adolescent Japanese girls following immunization with the human papillomavirus vaccine.** *Intern Med* 2014; 53(19): 2185-200.

- Researchers examined 40 adolescent girls to determine the underlying causes of several neurological conditions that occurred after HPV vaccination.
- Symptoms included headaches, dizziness, fatigue, limb pain, limb weakness, cold legs, menstrual disturbances, difficulty in standing up (orthostatic intolerance), fainting, tremors, gait disturbances, persistent asthenia, decreased memory, poor concentration and difficulty learning.
- Intradermal nerves showed abnormal pathology in the unmyelinated fibers.

161.

Brinth LS, Pors K, et al. **Is chronic fatigue syndrome/myalgic encephalomyelitis a relevant diagnosis in patients with suspected side effects to human papilloma virus vaccine?** *Int J Vaccines Vaccin* 2015; 1(1): 00003.

"We found that 87% and 90% of the patients fulfilled the diagnostic criteria for chronic fatigue syndrome/myalgic encephalomyelitis...and suggest that chronic fatigue syndrome/myalgic encephalomyelitis may be a suitable diagnosis for patients with severe and persistent suspected side effects to the quadrivalent HPV vaccine."

- Researchers examined 39 female patients who had symptoms compatible with autonomic dysfunction following HPV vaccination and found that most fulfilled the criteria for chronic fatigue syndrome/myalgic encephalomyelitis.

162.

Some girls develop premature ovarian insufficiency after HPV vaccination, which may affect childbearing

"Principles of informed consent, population health, and vaccine confidence require careful, rigorous and independent research to establish ovarian safety following HPV vaccination."

Little DT, Ward HR. **Adolescent premature ovarian insufficiency following human papillomavirus vaccination: a case series seen in general practice.** *Journal of Investigative Medicine High Impact Case Reports* 2014 Oct-Dec; 2(4).

- Current HPV vaccine safety research is inadequate to determine ovarian safety.
- This paper describes the case histories of three Australian teenagers who developed premature ovarian insufficiency following HPV vaccination.
- A diagnosis of idiopathic premature ovarian insufficiency in three adolescents following HPV vaccination has potential implications for future childbearing and reproductive health in young women targeted for the vaccine.
- Premature ovarian insufficiency can increase the risk of cardiac failure.
- Most women with premature ovarian insufficiency have an altered menstrual cycle as their initial symptom.
- Altered ovulation and menstrual patterns hasten the loss of bone density, which increases the risk for wrist and hip fractures in later life.
- Cohort studies of menstrual patterns in HPV-vaccinated and unvaccinated girls are essential, and should be conducted independent of commercial interests.

163.

The HPV vaccine may cause autoimmunity and ovarian failure

"We documented here the evidence of the potential of the HPV vaccine to trigger a life-disabling autoimmune condition. The increasing number of similar reports of post HPV vaccine-linked autoimmunity and the uncertainty of long-term clinical benefits of HPV vaccination are a matter of public health that warrants further rigorous inquiry."

Colafrancesco S, Perricone C, et al. **Human papilloma virus vaccine and primary ovarian failure: another facet of the autoimmune/inflammatory syndrome induced by adjuvants.** *Am J Reprod Immunol* 2013 Oct; 70(4): 309-16.

- In this paper, researchers analyzed the medical histories of three young women who developed secondary amenorrhea — the loss or suppression of normal menstrual flow — following HPV vaccination.

- These young women also experienced nausea, headache, sleep disturbances, arthralgia and several cognitive and psychiatric disturbances following HPV vaccination.

- Blood tests given post-vaccination suggest that the HPV vaccine triggered an autoimmune response.

- Post-vaccination autoimmune disorders are a major aspect of the autoimmune/inflammatory syndrome induced by adjuvants (ASIA). Several vaccines, including HPV, have been identified as possible causes.

- Based on the clinical features, the young women were diagnosed with primary ovarian failure, which also satisfied the criteria for ASIA syndrome.

164.

Clinical trials and marketing tactics by the HPV vaccine manufacturer may not be trustworthy

"The poor design of existing vaccine safety and efficacy trials may be reflective of the fact that in the past two decades the pharmaceutical industry has gained unprecedented control over the evaluation of its own products."

Tomljenovic L, Shaw CA. **Too fast or not too fast: the FDA's approval of Merck's HPV vaccine Gardasil.** *J Law Med Ethics* 2012 Fall; 40(3): 673-81.

- The HPV vaccine manufacturer aggressively influences public health policies despite obvious conflicts of interest.
- HPV vaccine advertising campaigns promote fear rather than evidence-based decision-making. Doctors must adopt an evidence-based approach in order to give their patients an objective assessment of vaccine safety.
- Coercive tactics such as vaccine mandates that are supported solely by vaccine manufacturers' own data is unacceptable.
- The HPV vaccine is neither safer nor more effective than Pap screening.

165.

Mello MM, Abiola S, Colgrove J. **Pharmaceutical companies' role in state vaccination policymaking: the case of human papillomavirus vaccination.** *Am J Public Health* 2012 May; 102(5): 893-98.

- Researchers interviewed 73 key informants in 6 states to investigate how the HPV vaccine manufacturer influenced health policymakers.
- The HPV vaccine manufacturer aggressively (and non-transparently) lobbied legislators to mandate their vaccine for school entry, drafted the legislation, provided the science, and made financial contributions to lawmakers.

166.

Published commentaries affirm that HPV vaccine safety and efficacy claims are at odds with factual evidence

"Whilst 12-year-old preadolescents are at zero risk of dying from cervical cancer, they are faced with a risk of death and a permanently disabling lifelong autoimmune or neurodegenerative condition from a vaccine that thus far has not prevented a single case of cervical cancer, let alone cervical cancer death."

Tomljenovic L, Shaw CA. **No autoimmune safety signal after vaccination with quadrivalent HPV vaccine Gardasil?** *J Intern Med* 2012 Nov; 272(5): 514-15. [Letter.]

- The HPV vaccine is unlikely to reduce cervical cancer rates beyond what Pap screening has already accomplished and offers no therapeutic benefits.
- Abundant evidence confirms that HPV vaccines can cause serious adverse events, including incapacitating autoimmune disorders and death.

167.

Tomljenovic L, Wilyman J, et al. **HPV vaccines and cancer prevention, science versus activism.** *Infect Agent Cancer* 2013 Feb 1; 8:6. [Letter.]

"Careful analysis of HPV vaccine pre- and post-licensure data shows that [efficacy and safety claims] are at odds with factual evidence and largely derived from significant misinterpretation of available data."

168.

Tomljenovic L, Shaw CA. **Who profits from uncritical acceptance of biased estimates of vaccine efficacy and safety?** *Am J Public Health* 2012 Sep; 102(9): e13-14. [Letter.]

"Careful scrutiny of Gardasil clinical trials shows that their design, as well as data reporting and interpretation, were largely inadequate."

Measles and MMR

Measles is a contagious disease that produces a rash all over the body. It is caused by a virus that affects the respiratory system, skin and eyes. Prior to the 1960s, most children caught measles. In developed nations, complications from the disease were unlikely. Previously healthy children usually recovered without incident. However, measles can be dangerous in populations newly exposed to the virus and in malnourished children living in undeveloped countries.

In the 1960s, a measles vaccine was introduced. In the 1980s, it was combined with vaccines for mumps and rubella into a single MMR shot. Although cases of measles declined after the measles vaccine was introduced, scientists now realize that childhood infections serve a valuable function and may be necessary for normal development of the immune system. For example, a large Japanese cohort study by Kubota and colleagues found that a history of measles and mumps in childhood is significantly protective against deadly heart attacks and strokes during adulthood. (Another study by Pesonen and colleagues, summarized in the next chapter, made a similar finding with chickenpox infections.)

Scientists also know that people who are vaccinated against measles can still contract the disease. In fact, an important paper by Rosen and colleagues provides strong evidence that measles can be transmitted from a fully vaccinated person to other fully vaccinated people. Other studies in this section confirm that loss of unsusceptibility to measles after MMR, and respiratory shedding of the virus, can allow the disease to spread, hindering the prospect of permanent long-term population-wide immunity.

Although some studies have not found a link between the MMR vaccine and autism, three studies in this chapter provide theories and evidence describing a possible link between MMR, autoimmune reactions and autism. Other studies confirm that children are significantly more likely to be rushed to an emergency room or admitted to a hospital during high risk periods after receiving MMR. For more studies related to measles and MMR besides those included in this section, read the chapters on allergies, seizures, thrombocytopenia, cancer and natural infections, and vitamin A, or use the index.

169.

Measles and mumps infections in childhood protect against deadly heart attacks and strokes during adulthood

"Measles and mumps infections were associated with decreased risks of mortality from cardiovascular disease."

Kubota Y, Iso H, et al. **Association of measles and mumps with cardiovascular disease: the Japan Collaborative Cohort (JACC) study.** *Atherosclerosis* 2015 Jun 18; 241(2): 682-86.

- This study investigated whether a history of measles and mumps during childhood alters the risk of dying from cardiovascular disease later in life.

- A lifestyle questionnaire, including a history of measles and mumps, was completed by 43,689 men and 60,147 women 40-79 years of age. They were followed for several years to determine their rates of mortality from atherosclerotic cardiovascular disease.

- Men who contracted measles in childhood were significantly less likely to die from total cardiovascular disease compared to men who were not infected with either measles or mumps (hazard ratio, HR = 0.92). Men who had mumps were significantly protected against dying from a stroke (HR = 0.52).

- Men who had both measles and mumps in childhood were significantly less likely to die from a myocardial infarction, that is, a heart attack (HR = 0.71).

- Women who had both measles and mumps in childhood were significantly less likely to die from total cardiovascular disease compared to women who had neither infection (HR = 0.83). They were also significantly protected against dying from a stroke (HR = 0.84).

- A history of measles and mumps decreases the risk of cardiovascular disease.

- The results of this study may be explained by the "hygiene hypothesis," which proposes that infections suffered during childhood are necessary for normal development of the immune system regulating T helper cells, Th1 and Th2, which control inflammation at the arterial wall leading to atherosclerosis.

170.

Measles can be spread from fully vaccinated people to other fully vaccinated people

"This is the first report in which a person with a verified secondary vaccine failure despite receipt of two doses of MMR was demonstrated to be capable of transmitting disease to other individuals."

Rosen JB, Rota JS, et al. **Outbreak of measles among persons with prior evidence of immunity, New York City, 2011.** *Clin Infect Dis* 2014 May; 58(9): 1205-10.

- Scientists know that people who are vaccinated against measles can still get the disease. However, they originally believed that only unvaccinated people can spread measles to others.

- This paper provides evidence that measles can be transmitted from a fully vaccinated person to other fully vaccinated individuals.

- A 22-year-old woman with documented evidence of having received two doses of a measles vaccine transmitted measles to four people who were supposedly immune. Two of the people were fully vaccinated against measles; the other two had documentation confirming prior measles antibody protection.

- The vaccinated woman who transmitted measles to other people had low neutralizing antibody titer after infection, which provides a biologically plausible rationale for her ability to spread the disease.

- Measles antibody levels are expected to decline over time. However, the loss of asymptomatic natural boosting that used to occur when measles freely circulated could affect population-wide immunity against the disease.

- Widespread measles vaccination reduced public exposure to the measles virus reducing opportunities to boost immunity among vaccinated people, which may contribute to waning antibody levels, loss of population immunity to measles, and an increased ability of vaccinated persons to transmit the disease.

171.

Measles vaccine failures cause outbreaks of the disease

"This outbreak raises important questions concerning the relative contributions of vaccine failure versus failure to vaccinate."

De Serres G, Markowski F, et al. **Largest measles epidemic in North America in a decade — Quebec, Canada, 2011: contribution of susceptibility, serendipity, and superspreading events.** *J Infect Dis* 2013 Mar 15; 207(6): 990-98.

- In 2011, there was a large measles epidemic in Quebec, Canada. Passive surveillance identified 725 cases, of which 678 occurred in one outbreak. This paper analyzed the details of this outbreak.

- Measles vaccination rates were high when the outbreak occurred: 97% of children had received 1 dose by 28 months of age and 90% had received 2 doses. Rates were even higher by the time children entered school.

- The person who initiated the large measles outbreak — the index patient — was vaccinated in childhood.

- During the outbreak, 21 infants contracted measles and 4 were hospitalized, but none had pneumonia or serious complications.

- In a school outbreak where vaccination status was known, 49% of all measles cases were in children who had received 2 doses of the measles vaccine. (About half of all measles cases were due to vaccine failures.)

- Passive surveillance significantly under-reported the number of measles cases that occurred in fully vaccinated people.

- The outbreak eventually ended without aggressive interventions to stop transmission.

- Waning immunity in adolescents who received 2 doses of a measles vaccine suggests that elimination of measles may not be possible even with a 100% vaccination rate.

172.

Loss of immunity after MMR, and viral shedding, could spread disease and prevent herd immunity

"If wild virus can be spread via individuals with subclinical infections, it is doubtful whether population immunity (herd immunity), which is necessary to eliminate the three diseases, can be attained in large populations."

Trier H, Rønne T. **Duration of immunity and occurrence of secondary vaccine failure following vaccination against measles, mumps and rubella.** *Ugeskr Laeger* 1992 Jul 13; 154(29): 2008-13. [Danish.]

- This paper describes a loss of immunity to measles, mumps and rubella that occurs with the elapse of time after MMR vaccination, permitting subclinical (asymptomatic) infections that could spread the three diseases to other people.

173.

Morfin F, Beguin A, et al. **Detection of measles vaccine in the throat of a vaccinated child.** *Vaccine* 2002 Feb 22; 20(11-12): 1541-43.

"In the case presented here, the vaccine virus was isolated in the throat, showing that subcutaneous injection of an attenuated measles strain can result in respiratory excretion of this virus."

- Fevers induced by measles vaccination are related to the replication and shedding of the live vaccine virus.

174.

Kaic B, Gjenero-Margan I, et al. **Spotlight on measles 2010: excretion of vaccine strain measles virus in urine and pharyngeal secretions of a child with vaccine associated febrile rash illness, Croatia, March 2010.** *Euro Surveill* 2010 Sep 2; 15(35).

- The measles vaccine virus is excreted from the throat and only molecular genotyping can distinguish between wild-type and vaccine-related disease.

175.

The MMR vaccine may be associated with brain autoimmunity and autism

"Over 90% of MMR antibody-positive autistic sera were also positive for MBP autoantibodies, suggesting a strong association between MMR and central nervous system autoimmunity in autism. Stemming from this evidence, we suggest that an inappropriate antibody response to MMR, specifically the measles component thereof, might be related to pathogenesis of autism."

Singh VK, Lin SX, et al. **Abnormal measles-mumps-rubella antibodies and CNS autoimmunity in children with autism.** *J Biomed Sci* 2002 Jul-Aug; 9(4): 359-64.

- Many autistic children have elevated levels of antibodies to the measles virus but not to other viruses.
- This study analyzed MMR antibodies and brain myelin basic protein (MBP) autoantibodies in the blood of 125 autistic children and 92 non-autistic children (the control group).
- MMR antibodies were found in 60% — and MBP autoantibodies were found in 56% — of autistic children. None were detected in the control group.
- An abnormal antibody response to MMR vaccination may be associated with autism.
- The authors of this study believe that a large number of autism cases may result from neurological symptoms due to an atypical measles virus infection following MMR vaccination.
- This study provides evidence of an association between MMR vaccination (especially the measles component), central nervous system autoimmunity, and the inception of autism.
- Vaccines are administered to healthy people, mainly children, so vaccine safety must be virtually absolute.

176.

MMR and other vaccines made with human fetal cells may be linked with rising cases of autism

"Rising autistic disorder prevalence is directly related to vaccines manufactured utilizing human fetal cells."

Deisher TA, Doan NV, et al. **Impact of environmental factors on the prevalence of autistic disorder after 1979.** *J Public Health Epidemiol* 2014 Sep; 6(9): 271-86.

- Some vaccines are manufactured using human fetal cell lines. Human fetal DNA fragments can induce autoimmune reactions. DNA fragments and retroviruses can provoke genetic mutations.

- This study was designed to investigate whether human fetal and retroviral contaminants in childhood vaccines are linked to autism.

- This large cohort study included all children born after 1969 in the USA, Western Australia, the United Kingdom and Denmark with publicly available vaccination records and who later developed a diagnosis of autistic disorder.

- Birth year change points — dates when a substantial rise in the incidence of autism occurred — corresponded with the introduction of vaccines that were manufactured with human fetal cells: MMR, varicella and hepatitis A.

- There were highly significant associations between the number of children vaccinated against chickenpox ($r^2 = 0.88$) and hepatitis A ($r^2 = 0.68$) — which were manufactured using human cell lines containing fetal DNA and retroviral contaminants — and the number of children diagnosed with autistic disorder.

- The increasing number of vaccines made with human fetal cell lines is exposing infants and children to human DNA and retroviral contaminants that are associated with rising cases of autism.

- Increased age of the child's father and revisions to the American Psychiatric Association's *Diagnostic and Statistical Manual (DSM)* are not primary triggers for the rising prevalence of autism.

177.

MMR contains human fetal DNA fragments that may be associated with autism and genetic mutations

"This study is one of the first laboratory and ecological studies conducted that has examined the relationship between human fetal cell line manufactured vaccines, cellular DNA damage, and the worldwide autism epidemic."

Deisher TA, Doan NV, et al. **Epidemiologic and molecular relationship between vaccine manufacture and autism spectrum disorder prevalence.** *Issues Law Med* 2015 Spring; 30(1): 47-70.

- This study utilized statistical methods, laboratory procedures, molecular biology and genomic analysis to evaluate the public health ramifications of inoculating children with vaccines that contain human fetal DNA residue.

- Some vaccines, such as MMR and hepatitis A, are made with human fetal cell lines that create final products containing residual human fetal DNA fragments and HERV-K retroviral contaminants that may cause autoimmune reactions and insertional mutagenesis.

- Residual DNA can be delivered to the nucleus of a cell. The potential for exogenous DNA to enter the nucleus of a cell and integrate into its genome is a well-established biological process.

- Fetal DNA fragments in MMR and hepatitis A vaccines are significantly higher than the residual DNA limit established by FDA guidelines.

- Ecological data indicates a potential link between vaccines manufactured with human fetal DNA and the autism epidemic.

- In Norway, Sweden and the U.K., there is an association between reduced MMR vaccination rates and lower prevalence of autism spectrum disorders.

- Vaccines can be manufactured in animal or plant-based cell lines avoiding the dangers of residual human DNA and retroviral contaminants.

178.

Emergency room visits are significantly more common in children who were recently vaccinated against MMR

"There are significantly elevated risks of primarily emergency room visits approximately one to two weeks following 12 and 18-month vaccination."

Wilson K, Hawken S, et al. **Adverse events following 12 and 18 month vaccinations: a population-based, self-controlled case series analysis.** *PLoS ONE* 2011; 6(12): e27897.

- This study analyzed the health records of 413,957 children to determine the risk of serious adverse events at 12 and 18 months of age following receipt of recommended vaccines.

- The incidence of emergency room (ER) visits or hospital admissions 1 to 17 days after vaccination (the risk period) was compared with the incidence 20 to 28 days after vaccination (the control period).

- Children were significantly more likely to be rushed to an ER or admitted to a hospital during the risk periods after vaccination at 12 months (relative incidence, RI = 2.04 on day 9) and 18 months (RI = 1.34 on day 12) than during the control periods.

- For every 100,000 children vaccinated at 12 months of age, 598 additional children had one or more ER visits (1 child for every 167 vaccinated).

- ER visits during the risk period were more likely to require medical aid for multiple conditions compared to ER visits during the control periods.

- Children were excluded from analysis if they received a second vaccination during the observation period (0 to 28 days after the first vaccination), or if they died.

- Although the number of ER visits or hospital admissions in the days preceding vaccination were much lower than during either the risk or control periods after vaccination, no statistical analysis was published.

179.

Young children have an increased risk of requiring emergency care after MMR; Girls have an even greater risk

"Our findings suggest that girls may have an increased reactogenicity to the MMR vaccine."

Wilson K, Ducharme R, et al. **Increased emergency room visits or hospital admissions in females after 12-month MMR vaccination, but no difference after vaccinations given at a younger age.** *Vaccine* 2014 Feb 26; 32(10): 1153-59.

- This study analyzed the health records of 548,422 children to determine whether the sex of the child has an effect on the incidence of emergency room (ER) visits and/or hospital admissions after childhood vaccinations.

- Male and female children 12 months of age were 35% more likely to require emergency care 4 to 12 days after receiving MMR (the at-risk period) than 20 to 28 days post-vaccination (the control period).

- Although males and females had a significantly increased risk of ER visits and/or hospitalizations 4 to 12 days after their 12-month MMR vaccinations compared to the control period (relative incidence, RI = 1.35), females had an even greater risk (relative incidence ratio, RIR = 1.08).

- For every 100,000 children vaccinated at 12 months of age, 192 additional adverse events/ER visits in females can be expected, compared to males.

- For both males and females, the top reasons for ER visits and/or hospital admissions after their 12-month vaccinations were otitis media (ear infection/inflammation), acute upper respiratory tract infection, viral infection and non-infective gastroenteritis and colitis.

- Some possible reasons that females have a greater risk than males of adverse events after MMR vaccination include, a) lower birth weight, b) fewer maternal antibodies against measles, c) greater vitamin A deficiency, and d) general physiological differences.

Chickenpox and Shingles

Chickenpox, or varicella, is a contagious disease caused by the varicella-zoster virus. Before a chickenpox vaccine was introduced, doctors recommended exposing children to the disease because it is generally benign in childhood and complication rates increase when it is contracted by teenagers or adults. Herpes zoster, or shingles, is a reactivation of the varicella virus. When people regain their health after contracting chickenpox, the virus remains dormant in the body. Later, when immunity weakens, the virus can become active again as shingles, causing a painful cluster of blisters and postherpetic neuralgia — severe and debilitating nerve pain that can persist for weeks, months or years.

The first study in this chapter found that a bout of chickenpox in childhood is significantly protective against coronary heart disease during adulthood. Each additional contagious disease contracted during childhood, such as measles, mumps or rubella, increased the protective effect against acute coronary events by 14%. Other studies provide strong evidence that immunity against shingles is strengthened by periodic exposures to the circulating varicella virus. In the pre-vaccine era, frequent encounters with cases of chickenpox boosted antibody protection against shingles. However, national chickenpox vaccination programs reduced cases of the disease which restricted opportunities to reinforce immunity and increased herpes zoster incidence rates. Chickenpox vaccination programs reduced cases of chickenpox but increased cases of shingles. Medical costs, pain, and suffering associated with shingles generally are much greater than with chickenpox. To address this problem, a shingles vaccine was introduced.

Studies also show that the chickenpox vaccine is becoming less effective as more people are vaccinated, requiring the addition of booster doses, which are neither cost-effective nor as protective as the immunologic boosting that occurred naturally in the community during the pre-vaccine era. Some children vaccinated against chickenpox still contract the disease. Children vaccinated against chickenpox are also contracting shingles. Some vaccinated children are developing shingles from the virus in the vaccine while others are getting it from the wild (natural) varicella strain. In addition, both the chickenpox and herpes zoster vaccines are associated with serious adverse reactions. For example, according to the shingles vaccine manufacturer, congestive heart failure and pulmonary edema occurred more frequently in recipients of the shingles vaccine compared to those who received a placebo. A recent study by Lai and Yew found that the shingles vaccine significantly increases the risk of developing arthritis.

180.

Chickenpox during childhood is protective against coronary heart disease such as angina pectoris and heart attacks

"Childhood contagious diseases had a protecting effect against coronary heart disease. The risk for acute coronary events decreased significantly with increasing number of childhood contagious diseases."

Pesonen E, Andsberg E, et al. **Dual role of infections as risk factors for coronary heart disease.** *Atherosclerosis* 2007 Jun; 192(2): 370-75.

- The "hygiene hypothesis" suggests that exposure to infections in childhood may be important for normal development of the immune system.

- This study compared 335 adult patients suffering from unstable angina pectoris and myocardial infarction (heart attack) with 355 controls to examine whether a history of childhood contagious ailments can affect the risk of acute coronary events.

- Adults who contracted chickenpox as children were significantly protected against acute coronary events (odds ratio, OR = 0.67).

- Each additional contagious disease contracted during childhood, such as measles, mumps or rubella, increased the protective effect against acute coronary events by 14%.

- This study also found that enterovirus, herpes simplex virus, and *Chlamydia pneumoniae* infections increase the risk for coronary heart disease.

181.

The universal chickenpox vaccination program is neither effective nor cost-effective and caused a dramatic rise in shingles

"Rather than eliminating varicella in children as promised, routine vaccination against varicella has proven extremely costly and has created continual cycles of treatment and disease."

Goldman GS, King PG. **Review of the United States universal varicella vaccination program: Herpes zoster incidence rates, cost effectiveness, and vaccine efficacy based primarily on the Antelope Valley Varicella Active Surveillance Project data.** *Vaccine* 2013 Mar 25; 31(13): 1680-94.

- The Centers for Disease Control and Prevention (CDC) sponsored and promoted studies that showed positive outcomes of varicella vaccination but opposed—and attempted to block—publication of findings that were critical of the varicella vaccination program.

- The CDC published and promoted studies on the incidence of herpes zoster (shingles) that had serious methodological limitations.

- Serious adverse events after varicella vaccination contribute to offsetting the benefits of varicella vaccination.

- As varicella vaccination rates increase, the vaccine becomes less effective against chickenpox, and shingles cases rise. This is due to a reduction in opportunities for natural boosts to immunity (exogenous boosts) which occur from exposure to people who are shedding the natural or wild varicella virus.

- Varicella vaccination cost-benefit analyses that were used to justify initiating a national vaccination program disregarded the significance of a) exogenous boosting, b) morbidity from serious adverse reactions to varicella vaccination, and c) morbidity from increasing cases of herpes zoster among adults.

- The varicella vaccination program has proven to be neither effective nor cost-effective.

182.

The chickenpox vaccination program is neither effective nor cost-effective

"Under universal varicella vaccination, there has been a vaccine-induced decline in exogenous boosting. We estimate universal varicella vaccination has the impact of an additional 14.6 million herpes-zoster cases among adults aged under 50 years during a 50-year time span at a substantial cost burden of 4.1 billion U.S. dollars or 80 million U.S. dollars annually."

Goldman GS. **Cost-benefit analysis of universal varicella vaccination in the U.S. taking into account the closely related herpes-zoster epidemiology.** *Vaccine* 2005 May 9; 23(25): 3349-55.

- Studies concluding that the varicella vaccination program is cost-effective fail to account for its adverse effect on the incidence of herpes-zoster.

183.

Goldman GS. **The case against universal varicella vaccination.** *Int J Toxicol* 2006 Sep-Oct; 25(5): 313-17.

"Scientific literature regarding safety of the varicella vaccine and its associated cost-benefit analysis have often reported optimistic evaluations based on ideal assumptions. Deleterious outcomes and their associated costs must be included when making a circumspect assessment of the universal varicella vaccination program."

184.

Goldman GS, King PG. **Vaccination to prevent varicella: Goldman and King's response to Myers' interpretation of Varicella Active Surveillance Project data.** *Hum Exp Toxicol* 2014 Aug; 33(8): 886-93.

"When the costs of the booster dose for varicella and the increased shingles recurrences are included, the universal vaccination program is neither effective nor cost-effective."

185.

Vaccinating children against chickenpox increases the risk of shingles in teenagers and adults

"We were able to observe the increasing incidence of herpes zoster (shingles), while the incidence of varicella infection (chickenpox) was declining."

Wu PY, Wu HD, et al. **Varicella vaccination alters the chronological trends of herpes zoster and varicella.** *PloS One* 2013 Oct 30; 8(10): e77709.

- Historically, the varicella virus caused chickenpox primarily in children then remained latent for many years until cellular immunity declined. The virus would then reactivate as herpes zoster in adulthood.

- This study analyzed the health insurance claims of 1 million people in Taiwan to determine trends in cases of chickenpox and shingles before and after introduction of a national chickenpox vaccination program.

- As more and more children were vaccinated against chickenpox — and the varicella virus was no longer widely circulating throughout society — the incidence of herpes zoster increased.

- After children were vaccinated against chickenpox, cases of shingles increased in teenagers and adults.

- When adults have regular contact with children who are infected with chickenpox, they experience exogenous boosts to their immunity which decreases their likelihood of developing shingles.

- National varicella vaccination programs diminish the amount of chickenpox virus circulating in the environment, thus limiting opportunities to reinforce immunity, increasing the incidence of shingles.

- Herpes zoster tends to affect females more than males.

186.

Adult exposure to children with chickenpox protects against shingles

"The results of this study suggest that vaccination of children against varicella could lead to a prolonged period of increased incidence of zoster among unvaccinated adults, as a result of fewer exogenous exposures to varicella-zoster virus."

Thomas SL, Wheeler JG, Hall AJ. **Contacts with varicella or with children and protection against herpes zoster in adults: a case-control study.** *Lancet* 2002 Aug 31; 360(9334): 678-82.

- Herpes zoster (shingles) often occurs in older adults. Complications include substantial morbidity and severe pain (postherpetic neuralgia).

- Adults who had chickenpox as children may gain immunity against shingles by coming into contact with children who are infected with the varicella virus. Conversely, childhood vaccination programs that reduce varicella could increase the incidence of shingles in adults.

- This study was designed to test the theory that close contact with ill children or the varicella virus provides protection against shingles.

- Adults who had many social contacts with children in groups, and frequent contact with ill children, were protected against shingles.

- Adults who had 5 or more contacts with people known to be infected with varicella were significantly protected against shingles compared to adults with no such contacts (odds ratio, OR = 0.29).

- Childcare work lasting more than 5 years provided significant protection against shingles (OR = 0.06). Contact with a few children living in the home also conferred strong protection against shingles (OR = 0.34).

- Contact with many healthy children or shingles cases was not protective.

- This study confirmed that regular exogenous exposure to varicella protects adults (who were previously infected with chickenpox) against shingles.

187.

The chickenpox vaccine program decreased cases of chickenpox but increased cases of shingles and lowered the age of infection

"As varicella vaccine coverage in children increased, the incidence of varicella decreased and the occurrence of herpes zoster increased."

Yih WK, Brooks DR, et al. **The incidence of varicella and herpes zoster in Massachusetts as measured by the Behavioral Risk Factor Surveillance System (BRFSS) during a period of increasing varicella vaccine coverage, 1998-2003.** *BMC Public Health* 2005 Jun 16; 5: 68.

- This study investigated the impact of widespread varicella vaccination in Massachusetts on the epidemiology of chickenpox and shingles.

- Between 1998 and 2003, chickenpox vaccination coverage among children 19-35 months of age increased from 48% to 89%. During this period, cases of chickenpox in all age groups declined by 79%.

- Between 1999 and 2003, the chickenpox vaccination rate among children 19-35 months of age increased from 66% to 89%. Cases of shingles in all age groups (including the elderly) increased by 90%, a highly significant trend. Cases of shingles in the 25-44 year age group significantly increased by 161%.

188.

Davies EC, Langston DP, et al. **Herpes zoster ophthalmicus: declining age at presentation.** *Br J Ophthalmol* 2015 Jul 15. [Epub ahead of print.]

"Our study suggests that varicella vaccination of children remains a possible explanation for the increased number of cases and reduction in mean age of newly diagnosed [herpes zoster ophthalmicus] patients."

- This study investigated 913 patients at a U.S. hospital diagnosed with herpes zoster ophthalmicus (HZO), severe and painful shingles of the eye. The number of cases at this hospital increased from 71 in 2007 to 195 in 2013. The mean age of HZO patients decreased significantly during this same period.

189.

The "success" of the childhood chickenpox vaccination program is causing an increase of shingles in adults

"A 100% effective chickenpox vaccine given to 1 year olds would cause a 1.75 times peak increase in herpes zoster 31 years after implementation. This increase is predicted to occur mainly in younger age groups than is currently assumed."

Ogunjimi B, Willem L, et al. **Integrating between-host transmission and within-host immunity to analyze the impact of varicella vaccination on zoster.** *Elife* 2015 Jul 11; 4: e07116.

- Researchers developed a mathematical model to simulate the effects of varicella vaccination on net increases in herpes zoster incidence.

190.

Jardine A, Conaty SJ, et al. **Herpes zoster in Australia: evidence of increase in incidence in adults attributable to varicella immunization?** *Epidemiol Infect* 2011 May; 139(5): 658-65.

- Cases of herpes zoster increased between 2% and 6% annually in Australian adults following a national chickenpox vaccination program for children.

191.

Goldman GS. **Universal varicella vaccination: efficacy trends and effect on herpes zoster.** *Int J Toxicol* 2005 Jul-Aug; 24(4): 205-13.

- The chickenpox vaccine is becoming less effective as more people are vaccinated, necessitating the addition of booster doses, which are neither cost-effective nor as protective as the immunologic boosting that occurred naturally in the community during the pre-vaccine era.

- The "success" of the chickenpox vaccine in reducing cases of the disease is causing increased cases of herpes zoster.

192.

Hospitalization rates due to severe cases of shingles, and annual hospital expenses for required care, increased significantly after the chickenpox vaccine was introduced

"The decrease in hospitalizations and charges for varicella-related hospital discharges was less than the increase in hospitalizations and charges for herpes zoster-related hospital discharges."

Patel MS, Gebremariam A, Davis MM. **Herpes zoster-related hospitalizations and expenditures before and after introduction of the varicella vaccine in the United States.** *Infect Control Hosp Epidemiol* 2008 Dec; 29(12): 1157-63.

- The varicella vaccine for chickenpox was introduced and recommended for U.S. children in 1995.
- This study was designed to determine the hospitalization rates due to severe cases of herpes zoster (as measured by herpes zoster-related hospital discharges) from 1993 through 2004, that is, before and after varicella vaccination was introduced and promoted in the United States.
- This study also measured the average annual hospital charges to health insurance companies for herpes zoster-related hospitalizations.
- Population-adjusted rates of herpes zoster did not change significantly from 1993 (before the chickenpox vaccine was introduced) through 2000 (the first few years after the chickenpox vaccine was introduced).
- In 2001, herpes zoster-related hospitalization rates started to rise and by 2004 were significantly higher than any of the rates during prior years.
- By 2004, hospital expenses for hospitalizations due to herpes zoster increased by more than $700 million annually.
- Adults 60 years of age and older accounted for 74% of the herpes zoster-related hospital expenses in 2004.

193.

Scientists knew that vaccinating children against chickenpox would cause an epidemic of shingles in adults

"Mass varicella vaccination is expected to cause a major epidemic of herpes-zoster, affecting more than 50% of those aged 10-44 years at the introduction of vaccination."

Brisson M, Gay NJ, et al. **Exposure to varicella boosts immunity to herpes-zoster: implications for mass vaccination against chickenpox.** *Vaccine* 2002 Jun 7; 20(19-20): 2500-7.

- This study found that when adults are exposed to children with chickenpox, they gain protective immunity against shingles. This boost to cell-mediated immunity is expected to last for about 20 years.
- Eliminating chickenpox in a country that is the size of the United States could cause 21 million new cases of shingles resulting in 5,000 deaths.

194.

Edmunds WJ, Brisson M, et al. **Varicella vaccination: a double-edged sword?** *Commun Dis Public Health* 2002 Sep; 5(3): 185-86.

"The impressive reduction in chickenpox incidence observed in the U.S. may be a double-edged sword, foreshadowing a correspondingly large increase in zoster over the next few decades unless other steps are taken to prevent this."

- The more successful that a chickenpox vaccination campaign is at reducing cases of the disease, the greater will be an increase in cases of herpes zoster.
- Following a childhood chickenpox vaccination program, a shingles epidemic in adults is expected to last for 30 to 50 years.
- Morbidity associated with each case of shingles is 10 times worse than for each case of chickenpox. This will have "serious consequences for public health, cancelling out the benefit of reduced varicella incidence."

195.

It's not ethical to increase cases of shingles in adults and the elderly by reducing cases of chickenpox in children

"Introducing a vaccination program could advance the health of one population group (children) at the expense of another (adults and elderly)."

Luyten J, Ogunjimi B, Beutels P. **Varicella-zoster virus vaccination under the exogenous boosting hypothesis: Two ethical perspectives.** *Vaccine* 2014 Oct 25; 32(52): 7175-78.

- This paper considers the ethical dilemma of vaccinating children to prevent chickenpox, which decreases opportunities for exogenous boosts to immunity that are essential to protect adults and the elderly from shingles.

196.

Kelly HA, Grant KA, et al. **Decreased varicella and increased herpes zoster incidence at a sentinel medical deputising service in a setting of increasing varicella vaccine coverage in Victoria, Australia, 1998 to 2012.** *Euro Surveill* 2014 Oct 16; 19(41): pii=20926.

"From 1998 to 2012, the age-standardized varicella incidence risk, estimated from medical consultations [by the National Home Doctor Service], halved while the age-standardized incidence risk of zoster almost doubled. Both changes were statistically significant."

- This study analyzed the effect that a national childhood varicella vaccination program had on the incidence of chickenpox and herpes zoster (shingles).

- Although cases of chickenpox significantly declined after health authorities in Victoria, Australia introduced a national childhood varicella vaccination program, cases of shingles significantly increased.

- The incidence rate of shingles in Victoria, Australia doubled in people under 50 years of age and tripled in adults 50-59 years of age within a few years after introduction of a national childhood varicella vaccination program.

197.

Children vaccinated against chickenpox are getting shingles from the virus in the vaccine

"Varicella vaccination of children has decreased varicella disease incidence, but introduced the occurrence of herpes zoster from vaccine-type virus."

Chun C, Weinmann S, et al. **Laboratory characteristics of suspected herpes zoster in vaccinated children.** *Pediatr Infect Dis J* 2011 Aug; 30(8): 719-21.

- Scientists have made laboratory confirmation that some vaccinated children are developing shingles from the virus in the vaccine.

198.

Weinmann S, Chun C, et al. **Incidence and clinical characteristics of herpes zoster among children in the varicella vaccine era, 2005-2009.** *J Infect Dis* 2013 Dec 1; 208(11): 1859-68.

"Vaccine-strain herpes zoster can occur after varicella vaccination."

- Children who are vaccinated against varicella to protect them from chickenpox are contracting herpes zoster (shingles).

- Some of the vaccinated children are getting herpes zoster from the wild (natural) varicella strain. Other vaccinated children are developing herpes zoster from the vaccine-strain of the varicella virus.

- The vaccine strain and wild strain of varicella might be in the process of genetically recombining to cause some laboratory-confirmed cases of herpes zoster in children who were vaccinated against chickenpox.

199.

The chickenpox vaccine in South Korea is relatively ineffective and is causing increased cases of the disease

"High vaccine uptake, the lack of upward age-shift in the peak incidence, and the high proportion of breakthrough disease, with almost no amelioration in disease presentation among vaccinated patients, strongly suggest that varicella vaccination has not been effective in preventing varicella in South Korea."

Oh SH, Choi EH, et al. **Varicella and varicella vaccination in South Korea.** *Clin Vaccine Immunol* 2014 May (21(5): 762-68.

- Health authorities conducted a case-based study, a case-control study, and an immunogenicity and safety study to assess the effect of varicella vaccination in South Korea.

- Despite a 97% varicella vaccination rate in 2011, the number of chickenpox cases reported to the Korea Centers for Disease Control and Prevention (KCDC) skyrocketed from 22.6 cases per 100,000 population in 2006 to 71.6 cases per 100,000 population in 2011.

- The case-control study provides evidence that the varicella vaccine is relatively ineffective in South Korea.

- A high proportion of children who were vaccinated against chickenpox still contracted the disease. The median time from varicella vaccination at 13 months of age to the onset of chickenpox was 3 years.

- Vaccinated children who contracted chickenpox did not have milder clinical symptoms than unvaccinated children who contracted the disease.

- Systemic adverse reactions occurred in 12% of the vaccinated children.

200.

The shingles vaccine can cause serious adverse events and its long-term efficacy is unknown

"The duration of protection beyond 4 years after vaccination with Zostavax is unknown."

Merck & Co., Inc. **Zostavax® (Zoster vaccine live), prescribing information.** Initial U.S. approval: 2006; revised Feb 2014.

- The shingles vaccine manufacturer summarized the clinical studies on safety and efficacy that were used to license its vaccine.

- A sub-study of the largest trial of the shingles vaccine found that serious adverse events occurred significantly more frequently in adults who received the shingles vaccine compared to those who received a placebo (RR = 1.53).

- Adults 80 years of age and older who received the shingles vaccine had serious adverse events at more than twice the rate of those who did not receive the vaccine (RR = 2.19).

- Serious cardiovascular events such as congestive heart failure and pulmonary edema occurred more frequently in recipients of the shingles vaccine compared to those who received a placebo. Respiratory infections and skin disorders were also more common in vaccine recipients.

- After the vaccine was licensed, additional adverse reactions were reported, including herpes zoster associated with the vaccine strain, arthralgia, myalgia, and anaphylactic reactions. Sensory loss and ophthalmic zoster were also more common in adults who got shingles after they received the vaccine.

- The vaccine is considered 51% effective in adults 60 years of age and older. However, recipients of the vaccine were followed for the development of shingles for as few as 31 days with a median of just 3.1 years.

- In elderly people 80 years of age and older, the shingles vaccine was unable to demonstrate that it is statistically more effective than a placebo.

201.

The shingles vaccine significantly increases the risk of developing arthritis, alopecia, and other serious adverse events

"Compared to the unexposed, patients with zoster vaccination had 2.2 and 2.7 times the odds of developing arthritis and alopecia, respectively."

Lai YC, Yew YW. **Severe autoimmune adverse events post herpes zoster vaccine: a case-control study of adverse events in a national database.** *J Drugs Dermatol* 2015 Jul 1; 14(7): 681-84.

- This study utilized the Vaccine Adverse Event Reporting System (VAERS) to investigate whether the herpes zoster vaccine is associated with severe autoimmune adverse events.

- Patients who received a herpes zoster vaccine were more than twice as likely to subsequently develop arthritis (OR = 2.2) or alopecia (OR = 2.7) compared to an unvaccinated control group.

202.

Fried, RE. **Herpes zoster.** *N Engl J Med* 2013 Oct 13; 369:1765-66. [Letter.]

"There was a 36% increase in the rate of serious adverse events associated with the herpes zoster vaccine in persons 60 years of age or older [compared to a control group]. The efficacy and safety of the herpes zoster vaccine in the elderly are questionable."

- For persons 80 years of age or older, the herpes zoster vaccine is not effective at preventing herpes zoster or postherpetic neuralgia and more than doubles the rate of serious adverse events.

203.

A new shingles vaccine contains $AS01_B$ — an adjuvant with unknown long-term effects

"Exacerbation or triggering of immune-mediated diseases in susceptible persons is a hypothetical concern for vaccines containing new adjuvants such as $AS01_B$ because of their immuno-stimulatory effects."

Lal H, Cunningham AL, et al. **Efficacy of an adjuvanted herpes zoster subunit vaccine in older adults.** *NEJM* 2015 May 28; 372: 2087-96.

- A phase 3 clinical trial of a new herpes zoster vaccine (called HZ/su) evaluated its safety and efficacy in adults 50 years of age and older.
- Vaccine reactions within 7 days occurred in 84% of vaccine recipients.
- Adverse reactions that prevented normal everyday activities occurred in 17% of vaccine recipients compared to 3.2% in the placebo group.
- Systemic reactions, including myalgia, fatigue, headache, shivering, fever and gastrointestinal symptoms, occurred in 66% of vaccine recipients.
- Systemic reactions that prevented normal everyday activities were more frequent after the second dose.
- A new adjuvant in this vaccine ($AS01_B$) has unknown long-term effects and may contribute to some of the systemic adverse reactions.
- Vaccine efficacy against herpes zoster was 97% in adults 50 years of age and older, with an average follow-up of 3.2 years.

Polio, Hepatitis B and Rotavirus

The studies in this chapter provide evidence of potential risks associated with polio, hepatitis B and rotavirus vaccines. In India, an aggressive polio vaccination campaign was followed by an epidemic of "non-polio acute flaccid paralysis" that is clinically indistinguishable from polio paralysis but twice as deadly. Some studies have found an increased risk of multiple sclerosis, chronic arthritis, and Guillain-Barré syndrome (GBS) after hepatitis B vaccination. Findings in other studies indicate the rotavirus vaccine may increase the risk of intussusception (life-threatening intestinal damage) and Kawasaki disease (a serious autoimmune ailment).

204.

Thousands of children were paralyzed following a polio vaccination campaign

"While India has been polio-free for a year, there has been a huge increase in non-polio acute flaccid paralysis. In 2011, there were an extra 47,500 new cases of non-polio acute flaccid paralysis. Clinically indistinguishable from polio paralysis but twice as deadly, the incidence of non-polio acute flaccid paralysis was directly proportional to doses of oral polio received."

Vashisht N, Puliyel J. **Polio programme: let us declare victory and move on.** *Indian J Med Ethics* 2012 Apr-Jun; 9(2): 114-7.

- This paper investigated the medical ethics of a polio eradication campaign in India that cost more than $2.5 billion and was followed by an exponential increase in cases of non-polio acute flaccid paralysis.

- In regions where children are vaccinated multiple times, the non-polio acute flaccid paralysis rate is up to 35 times higher than international norms.

- The non-polio acute flaccid paralysis rate in a given year correlates to the cumulative doses of oral polio vaccine received in the previous 3 years.

- Children who are stricken with non-polio acute flaccid paralysis have twice the risk of dying compared to those with a wild polio infection. (More than 43% of cases had residual paralysis after 60 days or died.)

- The significant increase in non-polio acute flaccid paralysis following India's aggressive polio eradication campaign was not investigated openly.

- Strain shifts of entero-pathogens induced by over-vaccination with the oral polio vaccine may be a factor in high rates of non-polio acute flaccid paralysis.

- It is not possible to extinguish polio because the sequence of its genome is known and scientists can resurrect it at any time.

- India's polio eradication campaign has been very costly due to the amount of human suffering and from a monetary standpoint.

205.

The hepatitis B vaccine significantly increases the risk of multiple sclerosis and other serious autoimmune diseases

"Chances of exposure to hepatitis B virus in adults is largely life-style dependent. Adults should make an informed consent decision, weighing the risks and benefits of hepatitis B vaccines, as to whether or not to be immunized."

Geier DA, Geier MR. **A case-control study of serious autoimmune adverse events following hepatitis B immunization.** *Autoimmunity* 2005 Jun; 38(4): 295-301.

- This study calculated the risk of serious autoimmune adverse events reported to the U.S. Vaccine Adverse Event Reporting System (VAERS) database after receipt of hepatitis B vaccination, compared to a control group that received a tetanus-containing vaccine instead.

- Adults who received a hepatitis B vaccine were 5 times more likely than the control group to develop multiple sclerosis (odds ratio, OR = 5.2).

- The hepatitis B-vaccinated group also had a significantly increased risk for rheumatoid arthritis (OR = 18), optic neuritis (OR = 14), lupus (OR = 9.1), alopecia (OR = 7.2), vasculitis (OR = 2.6), and thrombocytopenia (OR = 2.3).

206.

Le Houézec D. **Evolution of multiple sclerosis in France since the beginning of hepatitis B vaccination.** *Immunol Res* 2014 Dec; 60(2-3): 219-25.

"Figures in France show a definite statistical signal in favor of a causal link between the hepatitis B vaccine and multiple sclerosis."

- In France, cases of multiple sclerosis rose by 65% in the years following an aggressive national campaign to increase hepatitis B vaccination rates. This paper found a significant correlation between the number of hepatitis B vaccine doses given and the number of multiple sclerosis cases 1-2 years later.

207.

The hepatitis B vaccine triples the risk of developing multiple sclerosis

"These findings are consistent with the hypothesis that immunization with the recombinant hepatitis B vaccine is associated with an increased risk of multiple sclerosis."

Hernán MA, Jick SS, et al. **Recombinant hepatitis B vaccine and the risk of multiple sclerosis: A prospective study.** *Neurology* 2004 Sep 14; 63(5): 838-42.

- Some previous studies that evaluated a potential link between the hepatitis B vaccine and an increased risk of multiple sclerosis had significant methodological limitations.

- In this study, the General Practice Research Database (GPRD), containing comprehensive medical records from clinical practice in the United Kingdom, was utilized to compare 163 patients with a confirmed diagnosis of multiple sclerosis to 1,604 randomly selected controls.

- Patients with multiple sclerosis were 3 times more likely to have been vaccinated against hepatitis B within 3 years before the date of first symptoms when compared to controls who were not vaccinated (odds ratio, OR = 3.1).

- There was no increased risk of multiple sclerosis associated with tetanus and influenza vaccinations.

208.

Mikaeloff Y, Caridade G, et al. **Hepatitis B vaccine and the risk of CNS inflammatory demyelination in childhood.** *Neurology* 2009 Mar 10; 72(10): 873-80.

"The Engerix B (hepatitis B) vaccine appears to increase this risk, particularly for confirmed multiple sclerosis, in the longer term."

- Children with a confirmed diagnosis of multiple sclerosis were significantly more likely to have received the Engerix B brand of vaccine (OR = 2.77).

209.

Hepatitis B and rubella vaccines may cause chronic arthritis

"This study revealed that adult rubella and adult hepatitis B vaccines were statistically associated with chronic arthritis which persisted for at least one year."

Geier DA, Geier MR. **A one year followup of chronic arthritis following rubella and hepatitis B vaccination based upon analysis of the Vaccine Adverse Events Reporting System (VAERS) database.** *Clin Exp Rheumatol* 2002 Nov-Dec; 20(6): 767-71.

- The U.S. Vaccine Adverse Events Reporting System (VAERS) database was analyzed for any associations between adult rubella and hepatitis B vaccines and chronic arthritis.
- The risk of developing chronic arthritis was significantly higher in adults who received a rubella vaccine (relative risk, RR = 33) or hepatitis B vaccine (RR = 6.1) compared to adults who received a tetanus control vaccine.
- Chronic arthritis occurred primarily in females approximately 11 days after rubella vaccination and 16 days after hepatitis B vaccination.
- Chronic arthritis vaccine reactions may involve autoimmune processes.

210.

Pope JE, Stevens A, et al. **The development of rheumatoid arthritis after recombinant hepatitis B vaccination.** *J Rheumatol* 1998; 25(9): 1687-93.

"Recombinant hepatitis B vaccine may trigger the development of rheumatoid arthritis in...genetically susceptible individuals."

- Researchers investigated 11 people who developed rheumatoid arthritis after hepatitis B vaccination. All cases had persistent arthritis for more than 6 months, and all but 2 cases still had inflammatory arthritis 4 years later.

211.

Guillain-Barré syndrome (a neuromuscular disorder that can paralyze and kill) occurs after hepatitis B or influenza vaccination

"Our results suggest that vaccines other than influenza vaccine can be associated with Guillain-Barré syndrome (GBS). Vaccination-related GBS results in death or disability in one fifth of affected individuals."

Souayah N, Nasar A, et al. **Guillain-Barré syndrome after vaccination in United States: data from the Centers for Disease Control and Prevention/Food and Drug Administration Vaccine Adverse Event Reporting System (1990-2005).** *J Clin Neuromuscul Dis* 2009 Sep; 11(1): 1-6.

- Guillain-Barré syndrome (GBS) is an immune disorder that damages myelin sheaths of the nervous system, causing muscle weakness and paralysis.
- This study analyzed the Vaccine Adverse Event Reporting System (VAERS) to determine the rates and characteristics of GBS in the United States after receiving vaccinations.
- Between 1990 and 2005, there were 1000 cases of GBS reported in the United States after vaccination.
- In 77% of the cases, onset of GBS occurred within 6 weeks following vaccination.
- In 20% of the cases, vaccine-related GBS resulted in disability or death.
- In 63% of cases, GBS occurred following influenza vaccination, 9% of cases occurred after hepatitis B vaccination, and 27% of cases occurred after receiving other individual vaccines or combinations of vaccines.

212.

The rotavirus vaccine may increase the risk of life-threatening intestinal damage and Kawasaki disease

"The present study significantly associates RotaTeq vaccination with intussusception adverse events."

Geier DA, King PG, et al. **The temporal relationship between RotaTeq immunization and intussusception adverse events in the Vaccine Adverse Event Reporting System (VAERS).** *Med Sci Monit* 2012 Feb; 18(2): PH12-17.

- This study analyzed the Vaccine Adverse Event Reporting System (VAERS) to determine whether the rotavirus vaccine is associated with an increased risk of intussusception (severe and painful intestinal damage that can cause rectal bleeding requiring immediate medical attention).
- Adverse events that occurred after rotavirus vaccination were significantly more likely to be classified as serious, permanently disabling, requiring hospitalization, or were life threatening intussusception adverse events when compared to the total adverse events reported to VAERS.
- Onset of intussusception adverse events were significantly more likely to occur 3 to 7 days post-vaccination — a biologically plausible period — compared to other post-vaccination periods (risk ratio, RR = 2.7).

213.

Geier DA, King PG, et al. **RotaTeq vaccine adverse events and policy considerations.** *Med Sci Monit* March 2008; 14(3): PH9-16.

"These observations...raise serious questions regarding the use of RotaTeq in the US."

- Shortly after the rotavirus vaccine was introduced, 160 cases of intussusception and 11 cases of Kawasaki disease (a serious autoimmune ailment) were reported to VAERS, a significant increase over previous years.

Allergies

The studies in this chapter provide strong evidence that a) children who contracted measles were significantly less likely to develop allergies than children without a history of measles infection, b) children who contracted chickenpox were significantly less likely to develop asthma and allergies than children who were vaccinated against varicella, c) children who never received an MMR vaccine were significantly protected against allergies, and d) children vaccinated against pertussis were significantly more likely than unvaccinated children to be diagnosed with asthma, hay fever and food allergies.

214.

Children who contract measles are significantly less likely to develop allergies than children who are vaccinated against measles

"Our data suggest that measles infection may protect against allergic disease in children."

Rosenlund H, Bergstrom A, et al. **Allergic disease and atopic sensitization in children in relation to measles vaccination and measles infection.** *Pediatrics* 2009 Mar; 123(3): 771-78.

- This study investigated the health records of more than 10,000 children in five European nations to determine whether contracting measles or receiving a measles vaccine affects the risk of developing allergies.
- Children who contracted measles were significantly less likely to develop any allergic symptoms against common inhalant or food allergens (odds ratio, OR = 0.64) or to have been diagnosed with allergies by a doctor (OR = 0.51) than children who never contracted measles.
- Children who were vaccinated and never contracted measles were significantly more likely to develop rhinoconjunctivitis than children who were not vaccinated and never contracted measles (OR = 1.70).

215.

Shaheen SO, Aaby P, et al. **Measles and atopy in Guinea-Bissau.** *Lancet* 1996 Jun 29; 347(9018): 1792-96.

- This study investigated 262 young adults in West Africa to determine whether measles protects against atopy (an allergic reaction), defined by a positive skin-prick test to one or more of 7 allergens.
- Children with a history of measles were significantly less likely to have allergies than children who had been vaccinated and did not have a history of measles (OR = 0.36).

216.

Children with a history of measles are significantly less likely to develop allergies than children without a history of measles

"The results of this study indicate that findings of allergic disease are less frequent in children with a history of measles."

Kucukosmanoglu E, Cetinkaya F, et al. **Frequency of allergic diseases following measles.** *Allergol Immunopathol (Madr)* 2006 Jul-Aug; 34(4): 146-49.

- This study investigated the frequency of allergic diseases in children after they contracted measles as compared to children without a history of measles.
- Children who contracted measles were significantly less likely to exhibit sensitivity to dust mites that provoke allergic reactions or to require emergency treatment for asthma when compared to children without a history of measles.
- Children without a history of measles were significantly more likely than children with a history of measles to require inhaled corticosteroid (for the control of asthma).

217.

Kuyucu S, Saraçlar Y, et al. **Determinants of atopic sensitization in Turkish school children: effects of pre- and post-natal events and maternal atopy.** *Pediatr Allergy Immunol* 2004 Feb; 15(1): 62-71.

- This study analyzed 78 potential risk factors for 13 allergens in 1,144 Turkish children.
- A history of measles was found to be significantly protective against dust mite sensitivity.

218.

Children who contract chickenpox are significantly less likely to develop asthma and allergies than children who are vaccinated against chickenpox

"Wild-type varicella zoster infection up to 8 years of age has been shown to protect against atopic dermatitis and asthma."

Silverberg JI, Kleiman E, et al. **Chickenpox in childhood is associated with decreased atopic disorders, IgE, allergic sensitization, and leukocyte subsets.** *Pediatr Allergy Immunol* 2012 Feb; 23(1): 50-58.

- This study was designed to determine whether wild-type chickenpox infections protect against allergic disease.

- One hundred children up to 8 years of age who contracted chickenpox naturally (wild-type chickenpox) were compared to 323 randomly selected children who were vaccinated against chickenpox.

- Children up to 8 years of age who contracted wild-type chickenpox were significantly less likely than vaccinated children to develop asthma (odds ratio, OR = 0.12), allergic rhinoconjunctivitis (OR = 0.16), and atopic dermatitis (OR = 0.57).

- There was no association with food allergies.

- Children who contracted wild chickenpox also had significantly decreased total serum IgE levels compared with children who were vaccinated against chickenpox. (Serum IgE levels are elevated in people with allergic disease.)

- Compared to varicella-vaccinated children, wild-type varicella zoster infection decreased allergic sensitization by 89% (OR = 0.11).

219.

Children who never received an MMR vaccine were protected against allergies

"Prevalence of atopy is lower in children from anthroposophic families than in children from other families. Lifestyle factors associated with anthroposophy may lessen the risk of atopy in childhood."

Alm JS, Swartz J, et al. **Atopy in children of families with an anthroposophic lifestyle.** *Lancet* 1999 May 1; 353(9163): 1485-88.

- This study investigated the prevalence of atopy in children of families with an anthroposophic lifestyle. (Atopy refers to allergies. An anthroposophic lifestyle avoids vaccinations and antibiotics.)
- Scientists compared 295 anthroposophic children 5-13 years of age with 380 age-matched controls.
- Anthroposophic children had a significantly lower prevalence of allergies — less bronchial asthma, atopic dermatitis and allergic rhinoconjunctivitis — than controls (odds ratio, OR = 0.62).
- Children who never received an MMR vaccine had a significantly lower prevalence of allergies (OR = 0.67).

220.

Flöistrup H, Swartz J, et al. **Allergic disease and sensitization in Steiner school children.** *J Allergy Clin Immunol* 2006 Jan; 117(1): 59-66.

"Children having received measles, mumps, and rubella vaccination showed an increased risk of rhinoconjunctivitis, whereas measles infection was associated with a lower risk of IgE-mediated eczema."

- This study compared 4,606 anthroposophic children 5-13 years of age with 2,024 controls to determine factors that lower the risk of allergies.
- Children who received an MMR vaccine were more likely to develop rhinoconjunctivitis. Natural measles infection reduced the risk of eczema.

221.

Several children with a food-sensitive allergic skin disease had a clear improvement in their symptoms after they contracted measles

"Five patients with atopic dermatitis who were sensitive to hen's egg were observed before and after natural measles virus infection. Within 4 weeks of natural measles virus infection, the eczematous lesions clearly improved in four of the five patients in whom neither offending foods were eliminated, nor anti-allergic drugs, systemic steroids and steroid ointment administered."

Kondo N, Fukutomi O, et al. **Improvement of food-sensitive atopic dermatitis accompanied by reduced lymphocyte responses to food antigen following natural measles virus infection.** *Clin Exp Allergy* 1993 Jan; 23(1): 44-50.

- Children with food allergies and atopic dermatitis (dry, scaly, itchy skin rashes) had notable improvements in their symptoms after they contracted measles.

222.

Children who were vaccinated against pertussis or MMR were significantly more likely than unvaccinated children to be diagnosed with asthma and eczema

"In this observational study analyzing computerized primary care records, we found an association between MMR and DPPT vaccination and the incidence of asthma and eczema...."

McKeever TM, Lewis SA, et al. **Vaccination and allergic disease: a birth cohort study.** *Am J Public Health* 2004 Jun; 94(6): 985-89.

- This study examined the health records of 29,238 children between birth and 11 years of age to determine whether DPPT (diphtheria, polio, pertussis and tetanus) and MMR vaccinations affect the incidence of physician-diagnosed asthma and eczema.

- There was a very strong statistically significant association between exposure to DPPT or MMR and an increased risk of developing asthma and eczema. This link remained strong even after the authors adjusted for differences in how often vaccinated and unvaccinated children were taken to the doctor.

- DPPT-vaccinated children were 14 times more likely than unvaccinated children to be diagnosed with asthma (hazard ratio, HR = 14) and 9 times more likely to be diagnosed with eczema (HR = 9.4).

- MMR-vaccinated children were 3.5 times more likely than unvaccinated children to be diagnosed with asthma (HR = 3.5) and 4.6 times more likely to be diagnosed with eczema (HR = 4.6).

- After stratifying the children into smaller age groups and adjusting for fewer doctor visits by unvaccinated children — because children with fewer doctor visits have fewer opportunities to be diagnosed with allergies — the authors concluded that vaccinations are not a risk factor for allergic disease.

223.

Children who received a pertussis vaccine were 2 to 5 times more likely than unvaccinated children to be diagnosed with asthma

"The odds of having a history of asthma was twice as great among vaccinated subjects than among unvaccinated subjects."

Hurwitz EL, Morgenstern H. **Effects of diphtheria-tetanus-pertussis or tetanus vaccination on allergies and allergy-related respiratory symptoms among children and adolescents in the United States.** *J Manipulative Physiol Ther* 2000 Feb; 23(2): 81-90.

- This study examined whether there is an association between children who received a diphtheria-tetanus-pertussis or tetanus vaccine and subsequent allergies and allergy-related respiratory symptoms.
- Vaccinated children were twice as likely as unvaccinated children to be diagnosed with asthma and 63% more likely to be diagnosed with an allergy-related respiratory symptom in the past 12 months.

224.

Odent MR, Culpin EE, Kimmel T. **Pertussis vaccination and asthma: is there a link?** *JAMA* 1994; 272(8): 592-93. [Letter.]

- Researchers investigated 446 children (average age 8 years) who had been breastfed for more than one year and had received only breast milk in the first 6 months.
- Among the 243 children who received a pertussis vaccine, 10.7% were diagnosed with asthma, compared with 2% of the 203 children who were not vaccinated — a fivefold increase.

225.

Children who were vaccinated against pertussis were significantly more likely than unvaccinated children to develop asthma, hay fever and food allergies

"In the unvaccinated group, there were no significant associations between pertussis infection and atopic disorders. In the vaccinated group, all associations between pertussis infection and atopic disorders were positive."

Bernsen RM, Nagelkerke NJ, et al. **Reported pertussis infection and risk of atopy in 8- to 12-yr-old vaccinated and non-vaccinated children.** *Pediatr Allergy Immunol* 2008 Feb; 19(1): 46-52.

- This study evaluated an association between pertussis infection and allergic diseases by dividing 1,872 8-12-year-old children into two groups that were either pertussis-vaccinated or pertussis-unvaccinated in the first year of life.
- Pertussis-vaccinated children were more than twice as likely as pertussis-unvaccinated children to have asthma (OR = 2.24), hay fever (OR = 2.35) and food allergies (OR = 2.68).

226.

Kemp T, Pearce N, et al. **Is infant immunization a risk factor for childhood asthma or allergy?** *Epidemiology* 1997 Nov; 8(6): 678-80.

- In New Zealand, researchers investigated 1,265 children and discovered that of those who received diphtheria-tetanus-pertussis and polio vaccines, 23% had episodes of asthma while 30% had consultations for other allergic illness.
- Children who did not receive these vaccines had no recorded asthma episodes or consultations for allergic illness.

227.

Children who received their pertussis vaccines later than recommended were significantly less likely to develop asthma

"We have uncovered an association between timing of diphtheria-pertussis-tetanus (DPT) administration and onset of asthma at age 7 years. Delayed administration of the first dose of DPT of more than 2 months from the recommended 2-month period was associated with a reduced risk of childhood asthma by 50%."

McDonald KL, Huq SI, et al. **Delay in diphtheria, pertussis, tetanus vaccination is associated with a reduced risk of childhood asthma.** *J Allergy Clin Immunol* 2008 Mar; 121(3): 626-31.

- This study analyzed health records of 11,531 Canadian children to determine whether the timing of diphtheria-pertussis-tetanus (DPT) vaccination alters the odds of developing asthma by 7 years of age.

- Children are expected to receive diphtheria-pertussis-tetanus vaccinations at 2, 4, 6 and 18 months of age. In children whose first dose was delayed more than 2 months, the risk of developing asthma was reduced in half.

- The odds of developing asthma declined even further in children with delays in their first three doses.

- Asthma prevalence rates decreased significantly from 13.8% when the first dose was administered at 2 months of age to 10.3% when delayed until 3 months of age, to 9.1% when delayed until 4 months of age, to 5.9% when delayed beyond 4 months of age.

- Adjustments made for frequency of healthcare visits, the number of siblings, and family income did not alter the study findings.

228.

Children who received their pertussis, MMR or tuberculosis (BCG) shots later than recommended were significantly less likely to develop hay fever

"The odds of hay fever fall steadily with increasing lateness of vaccination for both DTP and MMR, and the tests for trend are significant. Postponement of routine immunization in early life is associated with a reduction in hay fever risk."

Bremner SA, Carey IM, et al. **Timing of routine immunisations and subsequent hay fever risk.** *Arch Dis Child* 2005; 90: 567-73.

- This study analyzed two large U.K. databases containing health records of more than 116,000 children to determine whether the timing of DTP, MMR and BCG vaccinations affects the subsequent risk of hay fever.

- Children who did not receive their third DTP shot until after their first birthday had a 40% reduced risk of developing hay fever compared to children who were vaccinated by 5 months of age as recommended (OR = 0.60).

- Children who did not receive their first MMR shot until after 2 years of age had a 38% reduced risk of developing hay fever compared to children who were vaccinated by 14 months of age as recommended (OR = 0.62).

- Children who received a BCG vaccine before their second birthday had a significantly increased risk of developing hay fever compared to children who never received it or received it later (OR = 1.34).

- Adjustments made for frequency of healthcare visits did not alter the study results.

Seizures

The studies in this chapter provide strong evidence that childhood vaccines significantly increase the risk of seizures. Children are nearly 8 times more likely to have epileptic events within 24 hours following their pertussis-polio-Hib vaccinations when compared to children who were not recently vaccinated. They are up to 6 times more likely to have convulsions 6 to 11 days after being vaccinated with MMR than at other times. Vaccine-related seizures and epilepsy syndromes are often non-febrile, severe and life-threatening.

229.

Childhood vaccines significantly increase the risk of seizures

"DTaP-IPV-Hib vaccination was associated with an increased risk of febrile seizures on the day of the first two vaccinations."

Sun Y, Christensen J, et al. **Risk of febrile seizures and epilepsy after vaccination with diphtheria, tetanus, acellular pertussis, inactivated poliovirus, and *Haemophilus influenzae* type B.** *JAMA* 2012 Feb 22; 307(8): 823-31.

- A population-based cohort study and a case series study of 378,834 children were undertaken to determine the risk of febrile seizures and epilepsy after receiving each of three recommended DTaP-polio-Hib vaccinations.

- Children vaccinated by the recommended schedule were nearly 8 times more likely to have febrile seizures on the day of their first vaccinations (hazard ratio, HR = 7.69), and 4 times more likely on the day of their second vaccinations (HR = 4.39), than children who were not recently vaccinated.

- The diphtheria, tetanus, acellular pertussis, inactivated poliovirus, and *Haemophilus influenzae* type B vaccines (DTaP-IPV-Hib) were given as a single combined shot, so it was not possible to determine which of the vaccines caused the febrile seizures.

- Children who received a pneumococcal vaccine along with their combination DTaP-polio-Hib vaccinations had significantly increased risks of febrile seizures on the days they received their first, second and third sets of vaccines and for up to 3 days after their second set of vaccines.

- Vaccinated and unvaccinated children had a similar risk of epilepsy after 15 months of age.

- Hazard ratios were adjusted for gestational age, birth weight, and parental history of epilepsy.

230.

Vaccinated children have a significantly increased risk of seizures

"This study suggests that there may be immunogenetic differences underlying vaccine-associated febrile seizures compared with other febrile seizures."

Tartof SY, Tseng HF, et al. **Exploring the risk factors for vaccine-associated and non-vaccine associated febrile seizures in a large pediatric cohort.** *Vaccine* 2014 May 7; 32(22): 2574-81.

- This study analyzed health records of 265,275 children aged 6 months to 3 years and compared vaccine-associated febrile seizures (those that occurred up to 15 days after any vaccine) with non-vaccine associated febrile seizures (those that occurred outside this period).
- Recently vaccinated children had a significantly increased risk of febrile seizures (RR = 1.63).
- Children with low one-minute Apgar scores had a significantly increased risk of vaccine-associated febrile seizures (RR = 3.40) but no increased risk for non-vaccine associated febrile seizures.
- African-American, Asian, and Hispanic children all had a significantly increased risk of febrile seizures versus White children.

231.

Principi N, Esposito S. **Vaccines and febrile seizures.** *Expert Rev Vaccines* 2013 Aug; 12(8): 885-92.

"Vaccine administration is the second leading cause of febrile seizures."

- Vaccines for pertussis, measles and influenza have been linked to febrile seizures.

232.

Vaccine-related seizures are often non-febrile, severe and life-threatening

"Vaccination-associated seizures present in the setting of various epilepsy syndromes, including severe childhood epilepsies, in greater than 10% of cases."

von Spiczak S, Helbig I, et al. **A retrospective population-based study on seizures related to childhood vaccination.** *Epilepsia* 2011 Aug; 52(8): 1506-12.

- This study was undertaken to describe the type and frequency of seizures and epilepsy syndromes in children after vaccination.
- A large German database of adverse events following vaccinations was analyzed for reported seizures and epilepsies in children 0 to 6 years of age.
- Of all confirmed seizures after vaccination, 15.4% were non-febrile.
- Of all children with confirmed epileptic events after vaccination, 12.6% exhibited various pediatric epilepsy syndromes, 11.7% were diagnosed with severe childhood epilepsies, and 8.5% presented with status epilepticus (a prolonged, life-threatening epileptic crisis).
- Epileptic events occurred on average 24 hours after receipt of inactivated vaccines and 7.5 days after attenuated vaccines.

233.

The MMR vaccine significantly increases the risk of seizures

"The rate ratio of febrile seizures increased during the two weeks following MMR vaccination."

Vestergaard M, Hviid A, et al. **MMR vaccination and febrile seizures: evaluation of susceptible subgroups and long-term prognosis.** *JAMA* 2004 Jul 21; 292(3): 351-57.

- This study analyzed data from 537,171 children to determine incidence rates of febrile seizures after MMR vaccination.
- Febrile seizures were nearly 3 times more likely to occur during the two weeks after MMR vaccination than at other times (incidence rate ratio, RR = 2.75).
- Siblings of children with a history of febrile seizures and children with a personal history of febrile seizures had significantly increased risk of seizures during the two weeks following MMR vaccination.
- Children with febrile seizures after MMR vaccinations had significantly increased risk of additional (recurrent) seizures compared with children who were non-vaccinated at the time of their first febrile seizure.

234.

Febrile seizures are serious adverse events that occur at significantly elevated levels after MMR vaccination

"This study confirms the known association between MMR vaccination and febrile convulsions."

Gold M, Dugdale S, et al. **Use of the Australian Childhood Immunisation Register for vaccine safety data linkage.** *Vaccine* 2010 Jun 11; 28(26): 4308-11.

- Researchers linked Australian childhood vaccination data with hospital data to confirm an increased risk of febrile convulsions 6-11 days after MMR vaccination.

235.

Miller E, Andrews N, et al. **Risks of convulsion and aseptic meningitis following measles-mumps-rubella vaccination in the United Kingdom.** *Am J Epidemiol* 2007 Mar 15; 165(6): 704-9.

"An elevated relative incidence of convulsion was found in the 6- to 11-day period after receipt of [MMR] (relative incidence = 6.26), consistent with the known effects of the measles component of MMR vaccine."

236.

Feenstra B, Pasternak B, et al. **Common variants associated with general and MMR vaccine-related febrile seizures.** *Nat Genet* 2014 Dec; 46(12): 1274-82.

"Febrile seizures represent a serious adverse event following measles, mumps and rubella (MMR) vaccination."

237.

The measles-mumps-rubella-varicella (MMRV) and MMR vaccines significantly increase the risk of seizures

"Providers who recommend MMRV should communicate to parents that it increases the risk of fever and seizure over that already associated with measles-containing vaccines."

Klein NP, Fireman B, et al. **Measles-mumps-rubella-varicella combination vaccine and the risk of febrile seizures.** *Pediatrics* 2010 Jul; 126(1): e1-8.

- The CDC-sponsored Vaccine Safety Datalink was used to compare the risk of seizures among 459,461 U.S. children 12-23 months of age who received the combination measles-mumps-rubella-varicella vaccine (MMRV) and those who received MMR and varicella vaccines (MMR+V) separately.
- Seizure risk was twice as high 7-10 days after MMRV than after MMR+V (relative risk, RR = 1.98).
- Children were nearly 8 times more likely to have seizures 8-10 days after vaccination with MMRV (RR = 7.6), 4 times more likely after MMR + V (RR = 4.0), and 3.7 times more likely after MMR alone (RR = 3.7), compared with seizure risk on other days.
- More than 90% of the seizures were acute and 87% were febrile seizures.

238.

O'Leary ST, Suh CA, et al. **Febrile seizures and measles-mumps-rubella-varicella (MMRV) vaccine: what do primary care physicians think?** *Vaccine* 2012 Nov 6; 30(48): 6731-33.

"After receiving data regarding febrile seizure risk after MMRV, few physicians report they would recommend MMRV to a healthy 12-15-month-old child."

239.

Children who receive MMRV have twice the risk of seizures compared to children who receive MMR and varicella vaccines separately

"We observed a notable increase in seizure incidence in the 7-10 days after either vaccine combination, which fits with the biologically plausible period for febrile seizures after a measles-containing vaccine."

MacDonald SE, Dover DC, et al. **Risk of febrile seizures after first dose of measles-mumps-rubella-varicella vaccine: a population-based cohort study.** *CMAJ* 2014 Aug 5; 186(11): 824-29.

- This study compared the risk of seizures among 277,774 Canadian children 12-23 months of age who received the combination measles-mumps-rubella-varicella vaccine (MMRV) and those who received MMR and varicella vaccines (MMR+V) separately on the same day.

- The incidence of seizures in the 42 days preceding vaccination was compared with the incidence of seizures during the biologically plausible "peak period" 7-10 days after vaccination.

- Children who were vaccinated with MMRV were 6 times more likely to have seizures 7-10 days after vaccination compared to the control period 42 days preceding vaccination (relative risk, RR = 6.57).

- Children who were vaccinated with MMR+V separately on the same day were 3 times more likely to have seizures 7-10 days after vaccination compared to the control period 42 days preceding vaccination (RR = 3.30).

- Children who were vaccinated with MMRV had twice the risk of seizures 7 to 10 days after vaccination compared to children who received MMR and varicella vaccines separately (RR = 1.99).

- Children who have febrile seizures are often rushed to the doctor or hospital for emergency care.

240.

Vaccination with MMRV (measles-mumps-rubella-varicella) significantly increases the risk of being hospitalized for febrile convulsions

"This study suggests a 2- to 4-fold increase in the risk of febrile convulsions in the interval 5 to 12 days after a first dose MMRV immunization compared to MMR immunization, and a 1.5 to 3.5-fold increase compared to MMR+V immunization."

Schink T, Holstiege J, Garbe E. **Epidemiological study on febrile convulsions after first dose MMRV vaccination compared to first dose MMR or MMR+V vaccination.** Presentation at the 57th Annual Meeting of the German Society for Medical Computer Science, Biometry and Epidemiology (GMDS), September 2012.

- This study analyzed the health records of 270,824 German children to determine the risk of being hospitalized with a diagnosis of febrile convulsions after vaccination with MMRV compared to vaccination with MMR or MMR plus varicella given separately on the same day.

241.

Schink T, Holstiege J, et al. **Risk of febrile convulsions after MMRV vaccination in comparison to MMR or MMR+V vaccination.** *Vaccine* 2014 Feb 3; 32(6): 645-50.

- German children were 4 times more likely to be hospitalized with febrile convulsions 5 to 12 days after vaccination with MMRV compared to children who received MMR (odds ratio, OR = 4.1), and 3.5 times more likely than children who received MMR+V separately on the same day (OR = 3.5).

242.

The DTP and MMR vaccines significantly increase the risk of seizures

"There are significantly elevated risks of febrile seizures on the day of receipt of DTP vaccine and 8 to 14 days after the receipt of MMR vaccine."

Barlow WE, Davis RL, et al. **The risk of seizures after receipt of whole-cell pertussis or measles, mumps, and rubella vaccine.** *N Engl J Med* 2001 Aug 30; 345(9): 656-61.

- Data from the CDC-sponsored Vaccine Safety Datalink (VSD) was analyzed to determine the risk of seizures among 679,942 children after vaccinations with DTP and MMR.

- Infants vaccinated with DTP were 9 times more likely to have seizures on the day of vaccination than infants not recently vaccinated (RR = 9.27). Children vaccinated with MMR were nearly 3 times more likely to have seizures 8 to 14 days after vaccination (RR = 2.83).

243.

Pruna D, Balestri P, et al. **Epilepsy and vaccinations: Italian guidelines.** *Epilepsia* 2013 Oct; 54 Suppl 7: 13-22.

"Diphtheria-tetanus-pertussis (DTP) vaccination and measles, mumps, and rubella vaccination (MMR) increase significantly the risk of febrile seizures."

Diabetes

The scientific papers in this chapter provide strong evidence that childhood vaccines significantly increase the risk of developing type 1 diabetes. In one study, children who received 4 doses of the *Haemophilus influenzae* type B (Hib) vaccine were significantly more likely than children who received no doses of the Hib vaccine to develop type 1 diabetes by 7 years of age. Other papers show an increased risk of developing type 1 diabetes after hepatitis B, MMR and pertussis vaccines. Epidemics of type 2 diabetes, obesity and metabolic syndrome have also been linked to vaccines.

244.

The Hib vaccine significantly increases the risk of developing type 1 diabetes

"Exposure to Hib immunization is associated with an increased risk of insulin dependent diabetes (IDDM)."

Classen JB, Classen DC. **Clustering of cases of insulin dependent diabetes (IDDM) occurring three years after *Hemophilus influenza* B (HiB) immunization support causal relationship between immunization and IDDM**. *Autoimmunity* July 2002; 35(4): 247-53.

- More than 240,000 children were split into three groups. One group received no doses of the *Haemophilus influenzae* type B (Hib) vaccine; another group received 1 dose; the third group received 4 doses of the Hib vaccine.

- At ages 7 and 10, the number of cases of type 1 diabetes in all three groups was tallied. At age 7, there were 54 more cases per 100,000 children in the group that received 4 doses of the Hib vaccine vs. the group that received no doses — a 26% increase. At age 10, there were 58 more cases per 100,000 children in the group that received 4 doses vs. the group that received no doses.

- Most of the extra diabetes cases occurred in statistically significant clusters 38 to 46 months after Hib vaccination, supporting a causal relationship.

- Mice that received Hib vaccines had an increased risk of developing IDDM.

245.

Wahlberg J, Fredriksson J, et al. **Vaccinations may induce diabetes-related autoantibodies in one-year-old children.** *Ann NY Acad Sci* 2003 Nov; 1005: 404-8.

- This paper provides evidence that vaccines contribute to alterations in the immune process that eventually may lead to type 1 diabetes.

- When analyzing the induction of autoantibodies, the titer levels of IA-2A (sensitive antibody markers associated with the development of type 1 diabetes) were significantly higher in children who received a Hib vaccine.

246.

Professional commentary substantiates a positive association between the Hib vaccine and type 1 diabetes

"The incidence of many other chronic immunological diseases besides diabetes — including asthma, allergies, and immune-mediated cancers — has risen rapidly and may also be linked to immunization."

Classen JB, Classen DC. **Public should be told that vaccines may have long term adverse effects.** *BMJ* 1999 Jan 16; 318(7177): 193. [Letter.]

- Vaccination against *Haemophilus influenzae* type b (Hib) starting after the age of 2 months is associated with an increased risk of type 1 diabetes.
- The increased risk of diabetes in Hib-vaccinated children is greater than the expected decline in complications from *H. Influenzae* meningitis.
- The public should be educated about long-term adverse effects of vaccines and demand proper safety studies prior to widespread vaccination campaigns.

247.

Classen JB, Classen DC. **Association between type 1 diabetes and Hib vaccine: causal relation is likely.** *BMJ* 1999 Oct 23; 319(7217): 1133. [Letter.]

- Distinct increases in diabetes have been documented in the United States and the United Kingdom after childhood Hib vaccination campaigns.
- Children who received 4 doses of the Hib vaccine were significantly more likely to develop type 1 diabetes by age 7 than children who received no doses of the Hib vaccine (relative risk, RR = 1.26).
- Data confirm a statistically significant causal link between the *Haemophilus influenzae* type b (Hib) vaccine and type 1 diabetes.
- The potential risk of the Hib vaccine exceeds the expected benefit.

248.

The hep B vaccine significantly increases the risk of developing type 1 diabetes

"Insulin-dependent diabetes mellitus (IDDM) is a common autoimmune disorder, and immune stimulation with a variety of immune stimulants has been associated with a rise in autoimmunity in both animals and humans. It is thus predictable that when you immunize a large population of children you would measure a significant increased risk for IDDM."

Classen JB. **Clustering of cases of IDDM 2 to 4 years after hepatitis B immunization is consistent with clustering after infections and progression to IDDM in autoantibody positive individuals.** *Open Pediatr Med J* 2008; 2: 1-6.

- This paper analyzed data from New Zealand, Italy and France confirming a significantly increased risk of IDDM associated with the hepatitis B vaccine.
- In New Zealand, the incidence of IDDM in children 0-14 years of age rose by 48% after a hepatitis b vaccination program was initiated. In Italy, hepatitis B-vaccinated children developed type 1 diabetes at a significantly higher rate than non-vaccinated children (RR = 1.40).
- In France, the incidence of IDDM in children 0-4 years of age rose by 61% after a hepatitis B vaccination program was initiated. A significant increase also occurred in children 10-14 years of age (RR = 1.31).
- There is a 2-4 year delay between hepatitis B vaccination and a rise in the incidence of IDDM, which is consistent with a causal relationship.

249.

Classen JB. **Diabetes epidemic follows hepatitis B immunization program**. *N Z Med J* 1996 May 24; 109(1022): 195. [Letter.]

- In 1988, New Zealand began vaccinating children against hepatitis B. Cases of type 1 diabetes skyrocketed from 11.2 cases per 100,000 children in the pre-vaccine years to 18.1 cases per 100,000 children in the post-vaccine years.

250.

Cases of type 1 diabetes increased after the introduction of MMR and pertussis vaccines

"The current findings indicate that there are clusters of cases of type 1 diabetes mellitus occurring 2-4 years post-immunization with the pertussis, MMR, and BCG (tuberculosis) vaccines."

Classen JB, Classen DC. **Clustering of cases of type 1 diabetes mellitus occurring 2-4 years after vaccination is consistent with clustering after infections and progression to type 1 diabetes mellitus in autoantibody positive individuals.** *J Pediatr Endocrinol Metab* 2003 Apr-May; 16(4): 495-508.

- This paper found sharp increases in the incidence of type 1 diabetes 2-4 years after the introduction of MMR and pertussis vaccines.

- A decline in type 1 diabetes occurred 3-4 years after pertussis and tuberculosis vaccines were discontinued.

251.

Classen JB. **The timing of immunization affects the development of diabetes in rodents.** *Autoimmunity* 1996; 24(3): 137-45.

"The timing and content of human vaccines can affect the development of diabetes."

- This study was designed to determine the effect of vaccines on the development of insulin-dependent diabetes in mice and rats.

- Injecting rodents with the pertussis vaccine starting at 8 weeks of life (rather than before 2 weeks of age) was linked with a higher incidence of diabetes.

- Clinical trials of new human vaccines are not designed to detect the development of insulin-dependent diabetes following receipt of those vaccines.

252.

The mumps vaccine may increase the risk of developing type 1 diabetes

"Mumps vaccination may not provide protection against diabetes mellitus, it may even provoke it."

Otten A, Helmke K, et al. **Mumps, mumps vaccination, islet cell antibodies and the first manifestation of diabetes mellitus type I.** *Behring Inst Mitt* 1984 Jul; (75): 83-88.

- Islet cell antibodies typically occur at the onset of diabetes in children and approximately 3 weeks after mumps infection, supporting a link between virus infections and diabetes.

- The mumps vaccine contains an attenuated live mumps virus, providing a plausible connection between mumps vaccination and diabetes.

253.

Quast U, Hennessen W, Widmark RM. **Vaccine induced mumps-like diseases.** *Dev Biol Stand* 1979; 43: 269-72.

- This paper investigated 16 cases of mumps and 2 cases of diabetes mellitus that occurred following mumps vaccination.

254.

Sinaniotis CA, Daskalopoulou E, et al. **Diabetes mellitus after mumps vaccination.** *Arch Dis Child* 1975 Sep; 50(9): 749-50. [Letter.]

- These researchers were among the first to document a case of childhood diabetes following mumps vaccination.

255.

All vaccines have the potential to induce diabetes; the risk may be even greater in families with a history of diabetes

"The results of this study are consistent with previous studies showing an association between vaccines and type 1 diabetes."

Classen JB. **Risk of vaccine-induced diabetes in children with a family history of type 1 diabetes.** *Open Pediatr Med J* 2008; 2: 7-10.

- This paper analyzed 11 years of health data to evaluate the link between childhood vaccinations and the development of type 1 diabetes.
- Vaccines for *Haemophilus influenzae* type b (Hib), MMR, polio, whole-cell pertussis, and the combined diphtheria-tetanus-inactivated polio vaccine were all associated with a significantly increased risk of type 1 diabetes.
- One dose of MMR increased the risk of diabetes by 88%. Two doses of the oral polio vaccine doubled the risk of diabetes (rate ratio, RR = 2.01).
- A child with a sibling who already has type 1 diabetes may be 70 to 150 times more likely to develop diabetes from a Hib vaccine than to benefit from it.
- All vaccines have the potential to induce diabetes.

256.

Classen JB, Classen DC. **Vaccines and the risk of insulin-dependent diabetes (IDDM): potential mechanism of action.** *Med Hypotheses* 2001 Nov; 57(5): 532-38.

"The current paper reviews multiple different mechanisms by which vaccines are known to manipulate the immune system and can induce an autoimmune disease such as type 1 diabetes."

- Many different vaccines, including live-virus and killed, have been linked to the development of insulin-dependent diabetes in humans and animals.

257.

There is a significant link between vaccine-induced type 1 diabetes and the autism epidemic

*"We have been publishing for many years that vaccine-induced inflammation is causing an epidemic of type 1 diabetes and other diseases. Our new data, as well as the extensive data from others regarding the role of inflammation in the development of autism, leaves little doubt vaccines play a significant role in the autism epidemic."**

Classen JB. **Prevalence of autism is positively associated with the incidence of type 1 diabetes, but negatively associated with the incidence of type 2 diabetes, implication for the etiology of the autism epidemic.** *Open Access Scientific Reports* 2013 May 20; 2(3): 679.

- This study analyzed the connection between autism prevalence in children of different races and the incidence of type 1 or type 2 diabetes.

- Races with the highest rates of type 1 diabetes generally had the highest rates of autism. Races with the highest rates of type 2 diabetes generally had the lowest rates of autism.

- There is a) a direct correlation between the incidence of type 1 diabetes and autism prevalence in children, and b) an inverse correlation between the incidence of type 2 diabetes and autism prevalence in children.

- Although this study did not calculate the effect of vaccines on type 1 diabetes or autoimmune autism, the direct correlation between these autoimmune diseases suggest they share the same pathophysiology and etiology.

- Simultaneous epidemics of type 1 diabetes and autoimmune/inflammatory autism are likely to have the same root cause.

* This quote was provided by the author in a press release — **Autism epidemic linked to epidemic of vaccine-induced diabetes** — published in *The Wall Street Journal* 2013, July 12.

258.

Epidemics of type 1 diabetes, type 2 diabetes, obesity, and metabolic syndrome have been linked to vaccines

"This paper describes two aberrant responses to immunization. At one extreme immunization leads to progressive autoimmune diseases including type 1 diabetes. A second response to immunization, and an opposite extreme to autoimmunity, is for the body to suppress the immune system through increased cortisol activity and other counter measures leading to type 2 diabetes and metabolic syndrome."

Classen JB. **Type 1 diabetes versus type 2 diabetes/metabolic syndrome, opposite extremes of an immune spectrum disorder induced by vaccines.** *Open Endocrinol J* 2008: 9-15.

- Metabolic syndrome is closely associated with type 2 diabetes in children and adults. It is defined by a collection of symptoms, including high blood pressure, obesity, cholesterol level abnormalities, and insulin resistance.

- This paper confirms a causal relationship between vaccination and metabolic syndrome using a) epidemiological evidence, and b) criteria set by Austin Bradford-Hill for establishing causation.

- Some people react to vaccines by developing autoimmune diseases such as type 1 diabetes while others develop type 2 diabetes/metabolic syndrome.

- Type 1 diabetes is an autoimmune disorder while type 2 diabetes is associated with obesity and insulin resistance. The inclination to develop either one is related to racial differences in cortisol secretions.

- There is a statistically significant correlation between the increasing number of vaccines given to children and childhood obesity.

- Vaccines are licensed based on small studies with brief followup. They are not designed to assess important safety issues such as metabolic syndrome.

259.

"Iatrogenic inflammation" (vaccination) caused epidemics of type 1 diabetes, type 2 diabetes, obesity, and metabolic syndrome

"Both the epidemics of type 1 diabetes and metabolic syndrome correlate with an increase in immunization."

Classen JB. **Review of evidence that epidemics of type 1 diabetes and type 2 diabetes/metabolic syndrome are polar opposite responses to iatrogenic inflammation.** *Curr Diabetes Rev* 2012 Nov; 8(6): 413-18.

- Metabolic syndrome is a cluster of symptoms — elevated blood pressure, high blood sugar, abnormal cholesterol levels, and obesity — that increase the risk of diabetes and heart disease.

- This paper reviews the evidence showing that epidemics of type 1 diabetes, type 2 diabetes, obesity, and metabolic syndrome in children are not only linked but are inverse responses to inflammatory illness induced by "iatrogenic inflammation" — medical intervention with vaccines.

- The likelihood of developing type 1 diabetes or type 2 diabetes/metabolic syndrome is linked to the release of cortisol, which is influenced by race.

- Poor diet and low exercise cannot explain the onset of metabolic syndrome in 6-month-old infants or why obesity protects against type 1 diabetes.

260.

Classen JB. **Italian pediatric data support hypothesis that simultaneous epidemics of type 1 diabetes and type 2 diabetes/metabolic syndrome/ obesity are polar opposite responses (i.e., symptoms) to a primary inflammatory condition.** *J Pediatr Endocrinol Metab* 2011; 24(7-8): 455-56.

- This paper provides additional evidence of a link between iatrogenic inflammation (vaccination) and concurrent epidemics of type 1 diabetes, type 2 diabetes, obesity, and metabolic syndrome.

261.

Epidemics of diabetes and inflammatory diseases are related to vaccine-induced immune overload

"Extensive evidence links vaccine-induced immune overload with the epidemic of type 1 diabetes. More recent data indicate that obesity, type 2 diabetes and other components of metabolic syndrome are highly associated with immunization."

Classen JB. **Review of vaccine-induced immune overload and the resulting epidemics of type 1 diabetes and metabolic syndrome, emphasis on explaining the recent accelerations in the risk of prediabetes and other immune-mediated diseases.** *J Mol Genet Med* 2014; S1:025.

- This paper discusses vaccine-induced overload and how it can explain many of the changes in epidemics of inflammation-associated disorders.

- Inflammation-associated disorders such as type 1 and type 2 diabetes, metabolic syndrome, autism, and autoimmune diseases have significantly increased in children following a significant increase in routine vaccinations.

- Vaccines are commercially designed to stimulate an immune response in children with the weakest immune systems. Thus, other children may have their immune systems over-stimulated, which increases the risk of inflammatory disorders and autoimmune diseases.

- Children are now being diagnosed with double diabetes, with symptoms of both type 1 and type 2 diabetes. Adults are being diagnosed with latent autoimmune diabetes in adults (LADA), or type 1.5 diabetes.

- Epidemics of inflammatory diseases have coincided with iatrogenic immune stimulation from vaccines.

- Safety trials for vaccine approval are either too short in duration or improperly use other vaccinated children as controls, which limit such studies from finding a link between vaccines and current epidemics of inflammation-associated disorders.

262.

The age when vaccinations are given can significantly influence the risk of developing type 1 diabetes

"These studies suggest that the timing of pediatric immunizations may alter the development of insulin-dependent diabetes mellitus (IDDM) in humans. The results also indicate that previous vaccine trials are flawed because they are not designed to detect associations between vaccination and autoimmune diseases, such as IDDM."

Classen DC, Classen JB. **The timing of pediatric immunization and the risk of insulin-dependent diabetes mellitus.** *Infect Dis Clin Pract* 1997 Oct 22; 6(7): 449-54.

- This paper linked vaccination schedules with health data in several countries to determine if there is a statistically significant relationship between the timing of vaccination and the development of type 1 diabetes.

- Nations that give the tuberculosis vaccine at birth generally have a lower incidence of diabetes than nations that give this vaccine to older children.

- In Finland, cases of type 1 diabetes increased by 147% in children 0-4 years of age after three new vaccines were added to the vaccination schedule.

- In New Zealand, there was a large increase in cases of type 1 diabetes after all children under 16 years of age were vaccinated against hepatitis B.

Thrombocytopenia

The studies in this chapter provide strong evidence that MMR vaccination significantly increases the risk of developing idiopathic thrombocytopenic purpura (ITP), a serious autoimmune disease that causes internal bleeding and can be life-threatening. Children are up to 7 times more likely to develop ITP within 6 weeks after MMR vaccination compared to the period prior to MMR vaccination. Children are also significantly more likely to develop ITP after receiving their pertussis, chickenpox and hepatitis A vaccines. Severe cases of ITP after vaccination can cause gastrointestinal and pulmonary hemorrhaging. In one study, ITP persisted for more than 6 months in about 10% of pediatric patients who developed the disease after vaccination.

263.

MMR significantly increases the risk of thrombocytopenia (ITP), a serious bleeding disorder

"The risk of idiopathic thrombocytopaenic purpura (ITP) occurring within 6 weeks after vaccination with MMR is significantly increased."

Black C, Kaye, JA, Jick H. **MMR vaccine and idiopathic thrombocytopaenic purpura.** *Br J Clin Pharmacol* 2003 Jan; 55(1): 107-11.

- Children were 6 times more likely to develop ITP within 6 weeks after MMR vaccination compared to children who were unvaccinated or not recently vaccinated with MMR (relative risk, RR = 6.3).

264.

Miller E, Waight P, et al. **Idiopathic thrombocytopenic purpura and MMR vaccine.** *Arch Dis Child* 2001 Mar; 84(3): 227-29.

"Our study confirms a causal association between MMR vaccine and idiopathic thrombocytopenic purpura (ITP)."

- Children 12-23 months of age were 6 times more likely to develop ITP 2 to 4 weeks after MMR vaccination than during a control period (relative incidence, RI = 5.80).

265.

Andrews N, Stowe J, et al. **A collaborative approach to investigating the risk of thrombocytopenic purpura after measles-mumps-rubella vaccination in England and Denmark.** *Vaccine* 2012 Apr 19; 30(19): 3042-6.

- This study found a statistically significant link between MMR vaccination and the risk of thrombocytopenic purpura (RI = 2.13).

266.

Thrombocytopenia, a serious autoimmune bleeding disorder, is 5 to 7 times more likely to occur after MMR vaccination

"Vaccines such as MMR may prompt immune thrombocytopaenic purpura (ITP)."

Rinaldi M, Perricone C, et al. **Immune thrombocytopaenic purpura: an autoimmune cross-link between infections and vaccines.** *Lupus* 2014 May; 23(6): 554-67.

- Immune thrombocytopenic purpura (ITP) is an autoimmune disease that causes internal bleeding and can be life-threatening, especially in children.
- ITP is 5 times more likely to occur after MMR vaccination (IRR = 5.48).

267.

Andrews N, Stowe J, et al. **Post-licensure safety of the meningococcal group C conjugate vaccine.** *Hum Vaccin* 2007 Mar-Apr; 3(2): 59-63.

"There was evidence of an increased risk of convulsions and idiopathic thrombocytopenic purpura following MMR vaccination."

- Researchers investigated 1,715 children admitted to a hospital with convulsions and 363 admitted with purpura (bleeding underneath the skin) to determine whether there was any epidemiological evidence that recent vaccinations increased the risk.
- Children were twice as likely to have convulsions 6 to 11 days after MMR (RI = 2.07) and 7 times more likely to develop ITP within 6 weeks after MMR (RI = 6.91) compared to the period prior to MMR vaccination.

268.

MMR, hepatitis A, varicella, and pertussis vaccines elevate the risk of internal bleeding

"The risk of immune thrombocytopenic purpura (ITP) after hepatitis A, varicella, and tetanus-diphtheria-acellular pertussis vaccine (Tdap) was significantly elevated in three discrete age categories."

O'Leary ST, Glanz JM, et al. **The risk of immune thrombocytopenic purpura after vaccination in children and adolescents.** *Pediatrics* 2012 Feb; 129(2): 248-55.

- Health records of 1.8 million children were analyzed to determine the risk of developing immune thrombocytopenic purpura (ITP) after vaccination. (Complications of ITP include intracranial hemorrhage and severe bleeding.)

- Researchers compared the incidence of ITP during the 42 days after vaccination with the incidence of ITP prior to vaccination and after the 42-day post-vaccination period. (Cases of ITP that occurred on the day of vaccination were excluded from analysis on the assumption that they were coincidental.)

- In children 12-19 months of age, ITP is 5 times more likely after MMR vaccination (incident rate ratio, IRR = 5.48). In children 11-17 years old, ITP is 12 times more likely after varicella vaccination (IRR = 12.14) and 20 times more likely after Tdap (IRR = 20.29). In children 7-17 years old, ITP is 23 times more likely after hepatitis A vaccination (IRR = 23.14).

269.

Bertuola F, Morando C, et al. **Association between drug and vaccine use and acute immune thrombocytopenia in childhood: a case-control study in Italy.** *Drug Saf* 2010 Jan 1; 33(1): 65-72.

"MMR vaccination was associated with an increased risk of developing immune thrombocytopenic purpura (ITP)."

- There is a significant relationship between children hospitalized for ITP and receipt of MMR within 6 weeks preceding hospitalization (OR = 2.4).

270.

Vaccines for MMR, pertussis, varicella, hepatitis A, hepatitis B, and influenza increase the risk of severe internal hemorrhaging

"A number of reports have clearly demonstrated that all of the live, attenuated viruses in the MMR vaccine can cause ITP whether administered alone or in combination."

Cecinati V, Principi N, et al. **Vaccine administration and the development of immune thrombocytopenic purpura in children.** *Hum Vaccin Immunother* 2013 May; 9(5): 1158-62.

- This paper summarizes studies documenting thrombocytopenia after MMR, pertussis, varicella, hepatitis A, hepatitis B, and influenza vaccinations.

- Severe cases of ITP after vaccination have been documented, including gastrointestinal hemorrhage, pulmonary hemorrhage, blood in the urine, serious bleeding requiring a blood transfusion, and surgery to remove the spleen.

- ITP after vaccination is most likely underreported because mild cases rarely elicit medical attention.

271.

Rajantie J, Zeller B, et al. **Vaccination associated thrombocytopenic purpura in children.** *Vaccine* 2007 Feb 26; 25(10): 1838-40.

- Researchers investigated pediatric patients who developed thrombocytopenia after vaccination. The bleeding disorder persisted in 26% of the patients for longer than 1 month and in 10% for longer than 6 months.

- The risk of thrombocytopenia after MMR vaccination is estimated to occur in 1 child for every 30,000 doses administered. (Most children receive 2 doses of MMR.)

272.

Several case reports describe thrombocytopenia after hepatitis B, DTaP, varicella and MMR vaccinations

"Vaccination may be a risk factor for infant thrombocytopenic purpura."

Hsieh YL, Lin LH. **Thrombocytopenic purpura following vaccination in early childhood: experience of a medical center in the past 2 decades.** *J Chin Med Assoc* 2010 Dec; 73(12): 634-37.

- This paper confirms cases of thrombocytopenia after hepatitis B vaccination at 1 month, DTaP at 2-3 months, varicella vaccination at 14 months and MMR at 16 months of age.

273.

Ronchi F, Cecchi P, et al. **Thrombocytopenic purpura as adverse reaction to recombinant hepatitis B vaccine.** *Arch Dis Child* 1998 Mar; 78(3): 273-74.

- This paper summarizes reports of thrombocytopenia after hepatitis B vaccination, excluding other causes.

274.

Neau D, Bonnet F, et al. **Immune thrombocytopenic purpura after recombinant hepatitis B vaccine: retrospective study of seven cases.** *Scand J Infect Dis* 1998; 30(2): 115-18.

- Seven cases of thrombocytopenia subsequent to hepatitis B vaccination are summarized in this paper. Alternate etiologies were excluded.

- Four of the cases had hemorrhagic manifestations.

- The mechanics of post-vaccinal thrombocytopenias are described.

Premature and Low Birth Weight Infants

The studies in this chapter provide strong evidence that vaccinating premature infants can cause heart and respiratory complications. After receiving vaccines, some premature infants are at risk of life-threatening apnea (temporary cessation of breathing). When premature infants are given several vaccines concurrently, they are 4 times more likely to have adverse cardiorespiratory reactions and 16 times more likely to have an abnormal C-reactive protein level (indicating inflammation or serious infection), compared to infants who are given a single vaccine. Preterm infants have immunological immaturities and should not always be vaccinated like full term infants. Full term infants with low birth weight have a significant risk of being rushed to an emergency room and admitted to a hospital after receiving vaccinations.

275.

Vaccinating premature infants can cause cardiorespiratory complications

"Our study revealed that some vaccines, including DTaP, even if administered alone, were associated with cardiorespiratory adverse events and abnormal CRP values in premature infants in the NICU. However, the incidence of these events was higher following simultaneous administration of multiple vaccines compared with administration of a single vaccine."

Pourcyrous M, Korones SB, et al. **Primary immunization of premature infants with gestational age less than 35 weeks: cardiorespiratory complications and C-reactive protein responses associated with administration of single and multiple separate vaccines simultaneously.** *J Pediatr* 2007 Aug; 151(2): 167-72.

- This study was designed to detect whether vaccinating premature infants causes cardiorespiratory events (episodes of apnea, bradycardia, or oxygen desaturation associated with cyanosis) and/or abnormal C-reactive protein (CRP) levels (indicating inflammation or serious infection).

- Cardiorespiratory events were noted in 16% of all vaccinated infants and 32% of those who received multiple vaccines simultaneously.

- Abnormal elevation of CRP levels occurred in up to 70% of those given a single vaccine and 85% of infants administered multiple vaccines.

- Infants who received multiple vaccines were nearly 4 times more likely to have vaccine-associated cardiorespiratory events and 16 times more likely to have an abnormal CRP value than infants who received a single vaccine.

- Vaccine-associated adverse reactions are not rare and may resemble serious infection in premature infants.

- Premature infants vaccinated at 2 months should be closely monitored for 48 hours due to the risk of cardiorespiratory events. Complications are more likely to occur with simultaneous administration of multiple vaccines.

276.

Adverse cardiorespiratory reactions are common in vaccinated premature infants

"We conclude that adverse cardiorespiratory events to primary immunization are common in very low birth weight preterm infants."

Meinus C, Schmalisch G, et al. **Adverse cardiorespiratory events following primary vaccination of very low birth weight infants.** *J Pediatr (Rio J)* 2012 Mar-Apr; 88(2): 137-42.

- Major cardiorespiratory events — apnea, bradycardia and desaturations — occurred in 35% of very low birth weight preterm infants after vaccination.
- Risk factors for adverse cardiorespiratory events after vaccination were low gestational age and respiratory support prior to vaccination.
- Despite awareness of predisposing factors, it is difficult to predict which infants will have an adverse reaction to their vaccinations, and how severe.

277.

Buijs SC, Boersma B. **Cardiorespiratory events after first immunization in premature infants: a prospective cohort study.** *Ned Tijdschr Geneeskd* 2012; 156(3): A3797. [Dutch.]

- Nearly 32% of vaccinated premature infants had cardiorespiratory reactions. Adverse reactions were more common in younger and lower weight infants.

278.

Flatz-Jequier A, Posfay-Barbe KM, et al. **Recurrence of cardiorespiratory events following repeat DTaP-based combined immunization in very low birth weight premature infants.** *J Pediatr* 2008 Sep; 153(3): 429-31.

- More than half (51.5%) of all vaccinated premature infants had an adverse cardiorespiratory reaction after their first vaccination, and 18% of these had a recurrence after their second vaccination.

279.

Major adverse reactions are common in premature infants who are vaccinated

"Vaccine-related cardiorespiratory events are relatively common in preterm babies. Problems were much more common if vaccine is administered at or before 70 days."

Sen S, Cloete Y, et al. **Adverse events following vaccination in premature infants.** *Acta Paediatr* 2001 Aug; 90(8): 916-20.

- This study assessed the frequency, severity and types of adverse reactions in very preterm infants following vaccination.
- Adverse reactions occurred in 38% of premature infants; 20% had major adverse reactions, including apnea, bradycardia or desaturations.
- Infants with major reactions were significantly younger and weighed less at the time of vaccination than babies who did not have major reactions.
- One-third (33%) of premature infants vaccinated at 70 days of age or less had major adverse reactions compared with none when vaccinated over 70 days of age.

280.

Faldella G, Galletti S, et al. **Safety of DTaP-IPV-HIb-HBV hexavalent vaccine in very premature infants.** *Vaccine* 2007 Jan 22; 25(6): 1036-42.

"Hexavalent (DTaP, inactivated polio, Hib and hepatitis B) immunization can cause apnea/bradycardia/desaturation in premature babies with chronic disease."

- Eleven percent of vaccinated premature newborns had adverse reactions.
- Nearly 22% of vaccinated premature newborns with chronic disease had adverse reactions.

281.

Premature infants should be monitored up to 72 hours after vaccination due to the increased threat of severe cardiorespiratory complications

"Cardiorespiratory monitoring of infants who are sufficiently preterm that they are receiving their first immunization prior to hospital discharge should be considered for 72 hours post-immunization."

Lee J, Robinson JL, Spady DW. **Frequency of apnea, bradycardia, and desaturations following first diphtheria-tetanus-pertussis-inactivated polio-*Haemophilus influenzae* type B immunization in hospitalized preterm infants.** *BMC Pediatr* 2006 Jun 19; 6:20.

- There is a substantial increased likelihood of adverse cardiorespiratory events in preterm infants after the first dose of vaccinations. Lower current weight is a risk factor.

- Vaccinated preterm infants were significantly more likely to have a resurgence of or increased episodes of apnea, bradycardia and blood oxygen desaturations than unvaccinated controls (odds ratio, OR = 2.41).

282.

Pourcyrous M, Korones SB, et al. **Interleukin-6, C-reactive protein, and abnormal cardiorespiratory responses to immunization in premature infants.** *Pediatrics* 1998 Mar; 101(3): E3.

"The frequency of cardiorespiratory difficulty and its occasional severity suggest a need to monitor premature infants for approximately 48 hours after routine immunization."

- Thirty percent of premature infants developed abnormal cardiorespiratory signs within 24 hours after vaccination.

- C-reactive protein and interleukin-6 values rose to abnormal levels in all but one infant after vaccination.

283.

Preterm infants who are vaccinated have a high risk for apnea and bradycardia

"For infants in the NICU without apnea during the 24 hours immediately before immunization, younger age, smaller size, and more severe illness at birth are important predictors of postimmunization apnea."

Klein NP, Massolo ML, et al. **Risk factors for developing apnea after immunization in the neonatal intensive care unit.** *Pediatrics* 2008 Mar; 121(3): 463-69.

- Pre-immunization apnea, lower birth weight (less than 2000 grams), and a younger age at time of vaccination (less than 67 days), are important predictors of post-immunization apnea.

284.

Schulzke S, Heininger U, et al. **Apnoea and bradycardia in preterm infants following immunization with pentavalent or hexavalent vaccines.** *Eur J Pediatr* 2005; 164: 432-35.

"Monitoring of all preterm infants following immunization in the neonatal intensive care unit is recommended."

- Recurrent or increased apnea or bradycardia occurred in 13% of respiratory stable preterm infants following receipt of combination vaccines.

285.

Clifford V, Crawford NW, et al. **Recurrent apnoea post immunisation: Informing re-immunisation policy.** *Vaccine* 2011 Aug 5; 29(34): 5681-87.

- Of preterm infants who experienced apnea after their initial vaccinations, 18% had recurrent apnea with subsequent vaccinations.

- Possible risk factors for recurrence included lower birth weight and ongoing hospitalization for complications associated with prematurity.

286.

Premature infants with very low birth weight or age are at risk for apnea and bradycardia after their vaccinations

"Apnea appeared significantly more often in children who were younger at the time of immunization."

Furck AK, Richter JW, Kattner E. **Very low birth weight infants have only few adverse events after timely immunization.** *J Perinatol* 2010 Feb; 30(2): 118-21.

- Apnea (temporary cessation of breathing) and/or bradycardia (an abnormally slow heart rate that cannot pump enough oxygen-rich blood to the body) occurred in 10.8% of very low birth weight infants after their vaccinations.
- When apnea occurred in preterm infants after their vaccinations, their chances of developing bradycardia also increased significantly (OR = 6.4).

287.

Sánchez PJ, Laptook AR, et al. **Apnea after immunization of preterm infants.** *J Pediatr* 1997 May; 130(5): 746-51.

- Smaller preterm infants of lower weight were the most likely to experience episodes of apnea and bradycardia within 72 hours after vaccination.

288.

Hacking DF, Davis PG, et al. **Frequency of respiratory deterioration after immunisation in preterm infants.** *J Paediatr Child Health* 2010 Dec; 46(12): 742-48.

- Some extremely low birth weight infants experienced apnea of sufficient severity following their vaccinations to warrant respiratory support.

289.

Preterm infants are at risk of life-threatening apnea after vaccinations

"When considering immunization for preterm infants, the benefits of early immunization must be balanced against the risk of apnea and bradycardia."

Botham SJ, Isaacs D, Henderson-Smart DJ. **Incidence of apnoea and bradycardia in preterm infants following DTPw and Hib immunization — a prospective study.** *J Paediatr Child Health* 1997 Oct; 33(5): 418-21.

- Preterm infants were monitored for 24 hours before and after they were vaccinated at 2 months of age. Only 1 of 98 preterm infants had apnea and/or bradycardia prior to vaccination compared with 17 of 98 after vaccination.
- Of the preterm infants who developed apnea and/or bradycardia after their vaccinations, 29% required respiratory support.

290.

Slack HD, Schapira D. **Severe apnoeas following immunisation in premature infants.** *Arch Dis Child Fetal Neonatal Ed* 1999 Jul; 81(1): F67-68.

"It is clear from our experience that some premature infants are at risk of life-threatening apnea after immunization."

- Premature infants who are vaccinated can develop severe apnea requiring resuscitation.

291.

Cooper PA, Madhi SA, et al. **Apnea and its possible relationship to immunization in ex-premature infants.** *Vaccine* 2008 Jun 25; 26(27-28): 3410-13.

- Several premature infants experienced apnea within 72 hours of receiving vaccinations.

292.

Preterm infants have immunological immaturities and should not always be vaccinated like full term infants

"Preterm infants have immunological immaturities that may impact on vaccine responses."

D'Angio CT, Hall CB. **Timing of vaccinations in premature infants.** *BioDrugs* 2000 May; 13(5): 335-46.

- Vaccines given to preterm infants do not always stimulate adequate immune responses that would normally be expected in full term infants.
- Sick premature infants may be susceptible to increased episodes of apnea after vaccination.
- Optimal care of preterm infants requires recognition that there are exceptions to the general rule that all preterm infants should be vaccinated just like full term infants.

293.

D'Angio CT. **Active immunization of premature and low birth weight infants: a review of immunogenicity, efficacy, and tolerability.** *Paediatr Drugs* 2007; 9(1): 17-32.

"Premature infants may have persistently lower antibody titers than full-term infants, even years after initial immunization."

- Premature infants have "immunologic immaturities" that may decrease vaccine efficacy.
- Sick premature infants have increased episodes of apnea or cardiorespiratory complications after their vaccinations.

294.

Vaccinating extremely low birth weight infants increases the risk of sepsis, respiratory support and intubation

"All extremely low-birth-weight infants in the neonatal intensive care unit had an increased incidence of sepsis evaluations and increased respiratory support and intubation after routine immunization."

DeMeo SD, Raman SR, et al. **Adverse events after routine immunization of extremely low-birth-weight infants.** *JAMA Pediatr* 2015 Jun 1.

- In this study, researchers evaluated 13,926 extremely low birth weight infants born at 28 weeks gestation or less to compare the incidence of sepsis evaluations, respiratory support, endotracheal intubation, seizures and death in the 3 days before and after vaccinations.

- Most of the infants (91%) received at least 3 vaccines between 53 and 110 days of age.

- The incidence of sepsis evaluations nearly quadrupled from the pre-vaccination to post-vaccination period (adjusted rate ratio, ARR = 3.7). The need for respiratory support (ARR = 2.1) and intubation (ARR = 1.7) also increased significantly in the post-vaccination period.

- Sepsis is a potentially fatal illness in which the body has a severe inflammatory response to an infection. Sepsis evaluations that yielded a positive blood culture result increased by 81% in the post-vaccination period compared with the pre-vaccination period.

- Five infants died within 3 days after receiving their vaccinations.

- The post-vaccination incidence of adverse events was significantly higher compared to the pre-vaccination period regardless of the type of vaccine, or combination of vaccines, administered.

- Lower gestational age infants had a significantly higher risk of sepsis evaluations and need for endotracheal intubation in the post-vaccination period, compared with older infants.

295.

Full term infants with low birth weight have a significant risk of being rushed to an emergency room and admitted to a hospital after receiving vaccines

"Lower birth weight appears to be correlated with an increased risk of emergency room visits within 24 hours of vaccination."

Wilson K, Hawken S, et al. **Impact of birth weight at term on rates of emergency room visits and hospital admissions following vaccination at 2 months of age.** *Vaccine* 2011 Oct 26; 29(46): 8267-74.

- This study investigated whether infants who are born full term but with low birth weight have an increased risk of adverse events following vaccinations at 2 months of age.
- The incidence of "emergency room visit and hospital admission" during the first 3 days post-vaccination was compared to a control period 9-18 days after vaccination.
- Emergency room visits occurred at a significantly increased rate in full term infants in the lowest birth weight group compared to those in higher birth weight groups (relative incidence, RI = 1.25) and when they were vaccinated before 60 days of age compared to after 60 days of age (RI = 1.57).
- Emergency room visits primarily occurred within the first 24 hours after vaccination.

Hexavalent Vaccines and Sudden Infant Death

Individual vaccines are often combined into one syringe to spare the child from multiple shots. For example, infants and young children in many European countries receive a series of hexavalent injections designed to protect against 6 different diseases: diphtheria, tetanus, pertussis, polio, *Haemophilus influenzae* type b, and hepatitis B. Although hexavalent injections may be more convenient for families, they might be less safe than other options.

The studies in this chapter provide strong evidence that hexavalent injections significantly increase the risk of sudden and unexpected deaths in young children. For example, in one study, children were 23 times more likely to die within 2 days after their fourth dose of a hexavalent injection, compared to the number of cases that would normally be expected. In another study, infants had a 2-fold increased risk of sudden infant death up to 2 weeks after the first dose of a hexavalent injection or following the co-administration of 6 individual vaccines.

Autopsies of children who died soon after receiving hexavalent injections showed unusual findings in their brains, including abnormal neuropathology. Parents and pediatricians should be aware that such fatalities are possible after hexavalent injections or multiple vaccines administered concurrently. (The Goldman and Miller study on page 17 also found that fatalities are possible after children receive multiple vaccines simultaneously.)

296.

Hexavalent vaccines significantly increase the risk of sudden and unexpected deaths in young children

"These findings based on spontaneous reporting...constitute a signal for one of the two hexavalent vaccines which should prompt intensified surveillance for unexpected deaths after vaccination."

von Kries R, Toschke AM, et al. **Sudden and unexpected deaths after the administration of hexavalent vaccines (diphtheria, tetanus, pertussis, poliomyelitis, hepatitis B, *Haemophilius influenzae* type b): is there a signal?** *Eur J Pediatr* 2005 Feb; 164(2): 61-69.

- Sudden deaths in young children shortly after they receive a hexavalent injection — 6 different vaccines in one syringe — have been reported. (The rationale for hexavalent vaccines was to reduce the number of injections that children receive to increase vaccination compliance and coverage.)

- This paper analyzed the risk of sudden unexpected death in young children within 1 to 28 days after receipt of a hexavalent vaccine.

- Standardized mortality ratios (SMR) were non-significantly higher than expected on the first day after receiving a hexavalent vaccine during infancy. In the second year of life, children were significantly more likely to die within 1 day (SMR = 31.3) or 2 days (SMR = 23.5) after hexavalent vaccination.

- These findings could not be attributed to limitations of the data sources, so there is a low probability they are chance coincidental.

297.

Hexavalent vaccines significantly increase the risk of sudden infant death

"In our study, only the first dose [of a hexavalent vaccine]...appears to carry a statistically significant increase in the risk of sudden infant death."

Traversa G, Spila-Alegiani S, et al. **Sudden unexpected deaths and vaccinations during the first two years of life in Italy: a case series study.** *PloS One* 2011 Jan 26; 6(1): e16363.

- This study was conducted to determine whether hexavalent vaccines increase the risk of sudden unexpected death in the first two years of life.

- There was a statistically significant 2-fold increased risk of sudden infant death 0-14 days following the first dose of a hexavalent product (rate ratio, RR = 2.2) or the co-administration of 6 antigens (RR = 1.9).

- There was a statistically significant increased risk of sudden infant death 0-7 days following the first dose of any vaccination (RR = 1.5).

298.

Kuhnert R, Hecker H, et al. **A modified self-controlled case series method to examine association between multidose vaccinations and death.** *Stat Med* 2011; 30(6): 666-77.

- This paper re-analyzed a previously published study on vaccines and sudden infant death using refined statistical methods.

- The re-analysis found that infants had an increased risk of sudden infant death within 3 days after receiving a second dose of a pentavalent or hexavalent vaccine (risk estimate = 2.56).

299.

Sudden deaths occur more frequently within a few days after hexavalent vaccines

"The Company evaluated whether the number of sudden deaths reported [after hexavalent vaccination] exceeded the number one could expect to occur by coincidence."

GlaxoSmithKline. **Biological Clinical Safety and Pharmacovigilance confidential report to regulatory authorities on Infanrix™ hexa (combined diphtheria, tetanus and acellular pertussis, hepatitis B, inactivated poliomyelitis, and *Haemophilus influenzae* type B vaccine), October 23, 2009 to October 22, 2011.** *GSK Confidential Summary Bridging Report* 2011 Dec 16: 246-49.

- A European hexavalent vaccine manufacturer produced a confidential evaluation on whether the number of sudden deaths reported following receipt of its combination vaccine exceeded the background incidence rate.

- Sudden deaths reported within 20 days after hexavalent vaccination were tabulated over a 2-year period. There were 67 sudden deaths reported within 20 days after vaccination during the first year of life and 8 sudden deaths reported within 20 days after vaccination during the second year of life.

- The manufacturer concluded that the number of sudden deaths reported after receipt of its hexavalent vaccine was below the number of cases expected.

- Despite the manufacturer's conclusion that its hexavalent vaccine does not increase the risk of sudden death, Table 36 on page 249 of the confidential report shows that 65 (97%) of the 67 sudden infant deaths occurred in the first 10 days after vaccination and just 2 deaths occurred in the next 10 days.

- Six (75%) of the 8 sudden deaths in children during their second year of life occurred in the first 3 days after vaccination.

- The manufacturer's conclusion was based on an *estimated* number of children actually vaccinated and failed to stratify by age within the two age groups.

- The confidential report was made publicly available by the Italian Court.

300.

Autopsies of children who died soon after receiving hexavalent vaccines confirm abnormal brain pathology

"Crude calculations of local epidemiology are compatible with an association between hexavalent vaccination and unusual cases of sudden infant death."

Zinka B, Rauch E, et al. **Unexplained cases of sudden infant death shortly after hexavalent vaccination.** *Vaccine* 2006; 24(31-32): 5779-80.

- This paper documented 6 cases of sudden infant death that occurred within 48 hours following the administration of a hexavalent vaccination.
- Autopsies of the children showed unusual findings in their brains, including abnormal neuropathology.
- There was a 13-fold increase in the risk of sudden death after hexavalent vaccination compared to an earlier period when the multi-dose vaccine was unavailable.
- Parents and pediatricians should be aware that such fatalities are possible after hexavalent vaccines.

301.

D'Errico S, Neri M, et al. **Beta-tryptase and quantitative mast-cell increase in a sudden infant death following hexavalent immunization.** *Forensic Sci Int* 2008 Aug 6; 179(2-3): e25-29.

"Clinical data, post-mortem findings...and laboratory analysis allows us to conclude that acute respiratory failure likely due to post hexavalent immunization-related shock was the cause of death."

- Scientists performed an autopsy on a 3-month-old infant who died within 24 hours of receiving a hexavalent vaccine and concluded that the multi-dose vaccination was the cause of death.

302.

Autopsies should be performed on all children who die suddenly after receiving vaccines

"This case offers a unique insight into the possible role of hexavalent vaccine in triggering a lethal outcome in a vulnerable baby."

Ottaviani G, Lavezze AM, Matturri L. **Sudden infant death syndrome (SIDS) shortly after hexavalent vaccination: another pathology in suspected SIDS?** *Virchows Archiv* 2006; 448: 100-104.

- In this paper, scientists document the case of a 3-month-old infant who died suddenly and unexpectedly shortly after being given a hexavalent vaccination (six vaccines in a single injection).

- Any case of sudden unexpected death that occurs soon after vaccination should undergo a full autopsy, including dissection of the brainstem and an examination of the cardiac conduction system, otherwise a true association between vaccination and death may escape detection.

303.

Matturri L, Del Corno G, Lavezzi AM. **Sudden infant death following hexavalent vaccination: a neuropathologic study.** *Curr Med Chem* 2014 Mar; 21(7): 941-46.

"We hypothesize that vaccine components could have a direct role in sparking off a lethal outcome in vulnerable babies."

- Scientists examined several sudden infant deaths that occurred within 7 days of hexavalent vaccination.

- The authors of this paper recommend that all sudden infant deaths occurring soon after hexavalent vaccination should be thoroughly investigated by an expert pathologist to objectively assess the possible role of the multi-dose vaccine in causing SIDS.

Cancer and Natural Infections

Several diseases have oncolytic (anti-cancer) properties. For example, tumor remissions after measles infection are well documented in the medical literature. Scientists have known for quite some time that infections in early life protect against various cancers in later life. Later born children have less cancer than first born children because they are exposed to more infections in early life from their siblings. Children who go to daycare in early life are more protected against cancers for the same reason. Vaccinations denied babies opportunities to become naturally infected, and with this reduction in exposure to disease there was a tradeoff — increased rates of cancer.

Numerous studies have confirmed a link between vaccinations and higher rates of cancer. Children who contract childhood ailments such as measles, mumps and chickenpox are significantly protected against various cancers later in life. Children who are vaccinated against childhood diseases are prevented from developing this anti-cancer protection. They are trading a reduced risk of infections for an increased risk of developing cancer later in childhood or as an adult.

The studies in this chapter provide strong evidence that infections protect against cancer while vaccines — which are designed to prevent infections — increased cancer rates. For example, Newhouse found that women who contracted mumps, measles, rubella or chickenpox had a statistically significant reduction in the risk of developing ovarian cancer. Kölmel found that individuals who contracted influenza, measles, mumps or chickenpox had a decreased risk of developing skin cancer later in life. Other researchers found that people with a history of chickenpox or influenza are significantly protected against brain tumors.

Albonico found that adults are significantly protected against non-breast cancers — genital, prostate, gastrointestinal, skin, lung, ear-nose-throat, and others — if they contracted measles, rubella or chickenpox earlier in life. Montella found that contracting measles in childhood reduces the risk of developing lymphatic cancer in adulthood. Alexander found that infection with measles during childhood is significantly protective — it cuts the risk in half — against developing Hodgkin's disease. Glaser also found that lymph cancer is significantly more likely in adults who were not infected with measles, mumps or rubella in childhood.

Gilham found that infants with the least exposure to common infections have the greatest risk of developing childhood leukemia. Urayama also found that early exposure to infections is protective against leukemia. Other studies confirm that children who receive MMR, pertussis or hepatitis B vaccines have a significantly elevated risk of developing leukemia.

304.

Women who contracted mumps in childhood were significantly less likely to develop ovarian cancer as adults

"The benign controls gave a history of mumps parotitis far more often than did the patients with ovarian malignancies. A causal association with a possible protective value is suggested."

West RO. **Epidemiologic study of malignancies of the ovaries.** *Cancer* 1966; 19: 1001-07.

- This study compared 97 women with ovarian malignancies to 97 women with benign ovarian tumors. Several variables were analyzed to determine if there were any significant differences between the two groups.

- Women with benign ovarian tumors were statistically more likely than women with ovarian malignancies to have contracted mumps earlier in life.

305.

Menczer J, Modan M, et al. **Possible role of mumps virus in the etiology of ovarian cancer.** *Cancer* 1979 Apr; 43(4): 1375-79.

- This study compared mumps antibody levels in 84 women with ovarian cancer to 84 women with non-malignant health conditions.

- Both groups had similar infection rates as indicated by serological evidence, but the women with ovarian cancer had 1) lower mumps antibody titers, and 2) a lower rate of clinical mumps history, suggesting that they had subclinical mumps (asymptomatic).

- Subclinical mumps — in contrast to symptomatic mumps — may be related to immune incompetence that permits the development of ovarian cancer.

306.

A mumps infection — but not mumps vaccination — protects women against ovarian cancer

"Our study suggests...unanticipated long-term anti-cancer benefits of a mumps infection."

Cramer DW, Vitonis AF, et al. **Mumps and ovarian cancer: modern interpretation of an historic association.** *Cancer Causes Control* 2010 Aug; 21(8): 1193-1201.

- Scientists obtained the blood of 161 women with mumps and 194 healthy controls to determine whether mumps provides immunity against ovarian cancer by producing anti-cancer antibodies against an abnormally expressed glycoprotein, MUC1.

- Scientists also conducted a meta-analysis of all published studies concerning mumps and ovarian cancer.

- This study found that anti-cancer (MUC1) antibodies in women infected with symptomatic mumps are significantly higher when compared to women without an active case of the disease.

- Pooled results from the meta-analysis of all pertinent studies found that women with a history of mumps had a 19% reduction in the risk of ovarian cancer (odds ratio, OR = 0.81).

- Mumps vaccination only creates anti-mumps antibodies, not anti-cancer protection, which requires an actual infection with symptomatic mumps.

- From 1978 to 1998, rates of endometrioid and clear cell tumors increased among white females. These are the types of ovarian cancer most strongly linked to and protected by anti-cancer antibodies produced by natural mumps infection (suppressed by increasing rates of vaccination during this period).

- This study provides the first biologically plausible explanation showing how mumps infection — but not mumps vaccination — provides immunity against MUC1, a cancer-related glycoprotein.

307.

Women with prior infections of mumps, measles, rubella or chickenpox were significantly less likely to develop ovarian cancer

"In our patients, two protective factors against ovarian carcinoma appear to be operative, a history of pregnancy and of infection by mumps, measles, rubella, or chickenpox."

Newhouse ML, Pearson RM, et al. **A case control study of carcinoma of the ovary.** *Br J Prev Soc Med* 1977 Sep; 31(3): 148-53.

- Scientists compared 300 women diagnosed with ovarian cancer to 300 women hospitalized with a gynecological condition other than ovarian cancer, and to another control group comprised of 300 women living in the same neighborhoods as the ovarian cancer patients.

- Compared to women in the control groups, fewer women with ovarian cancer could recall having been infected with mumps, measles, rubella or chickenpox.

- A history of having contracted mumps, measles, rubella or chickenpox was associated with a statistically significant reduction — 39%, 53%, 38% and 34%, respectively — in the relative risk of developing ovarian cancer.

- The relative risk of developing ovarian cancer was significantly reduced in women with a positive history of mumps (RR = 0.61), measles (RR = 0.47), rubella (RR = 0.62) or chickenpox (RR = 0.66).

- A history of pregnancy and the use of oral contraceptives also showed significant protective effects against ovarian cancer.

308.

Adults with previous infections of influenza, measles, mumps or chickenpox are less likely to develop malignant melanoma

"The study confirms the hypothesis that an inverse relationship exists between febrile infections and malignant melanoma...."

Kölmel KF, Gefeller O, et al. **Febrile infections and malignant melanoma: results of a case-control study.** *Melanoma Res* 1992; 2(3): 207-11.

- This study compared 139 hospitalized melanoma patients with 271 controls to determine whether febrile infections provide natural immunity against skin cancer (malignant melanoma).
- Individuals who contracted measles, mumps or chickenpox in childhood had a decreased risk of developing melanoma later in life.
- Adults were significantly protected against malignant melanoma if they had a chronic infectious disease (OR = 0.32) an infectious wound (OR = 0.21), or if they contracted influenza during the previous 5-year period (OR = 0.32).
- Adults with two or more febrile infections during the previous 5-year period were substantially less likely to develop malignant melanoma when compared to adults with no febrile infections during this period (OR = 0.20).

309.

Kölmel KF, Pfahlberg A, et al. **Infections and melanoma risk: results of a multicentre EORTC case-control study. European Organization for Research and Treatment of Cancer.** *Melanoma Res* 1999; 9(5): 511-19.

- This study compared the history of severe infections in 603 European and Israeli melanoma patients with that of 627 population controls.
- Significant reductions in melanoma risk were found with nearly all infections, including influenza (OR = 0.65) and pneumonia (OR = 0.45). Higher fevers and an increasing number of infections also reduced the risk of melanoma.

310.

Infectious diseases, including chickenpox and influenza, significantly reduce the risk of developing a brain tumor

"In this report, we present serologic support for the finding that glioma cases were less likely than controls either to have had varicella-zoster infection or to have antibodies to this virus."

Wrensch M, Weinberg A, et al. **Does prior infection with varicella-zoster virus influence risk of adult glioma?** *Am J Epidemiol* 1997 Apr 1; 145(7): 594-97.

- Scientists compared 381 adults with glioma (brain tumors) to 414 gender-, age-, and ethnicity-matched controls to determine whether having a history of varicella-zoster virus infection reduces the risk of developing a glioma.

- Adults with glioma were significantly less likely than controls to report a history of chickenpox (OR = 0.40) or shingles (OR = 0.50).

- Blood tests measuring antibodies to the varicella-zoster virus confirmed that glioma cases were less likely than controls to have had chickenpox.

311.

Schlehofer B, Blettner M, et al. **Role of medical history in brain tumour development. Results from the international adult brain tumour study**. *Int J Cancer* 1999 Jul 19; 82(2): 155-60.

"The decreased risks for glioma in subjects reporting a history of...infectious diseases may indicate an influence of immunological factors on the development of glioma."

- Scientists compared 1,509 brain tumor patients from six countries to 2,493 controls to determine if certain medical conditions cause brain tumors.

- Individuals who reported a history of infectious diseases, including influenza, had a 28% reduction in the risk of developing glioma (OR = 0.72).

312.

Wild chickenpox infections protect against brain tumors

"Statistically significant inverse associations of adult glioma with history of chickenpox and immunoglobulin G antibodies to varicella-zoster virus have been reported."

Wrensch M, Weinberg A, et al. **History of chickenpox and shingles and prevalence of antibodies to varicella-zoster virus and three other herpesviruses among adults with glioma and controls.** *Am J Epidemiol* 2005 May 15; 161(10): 929-38.

- This study compared 229 adults with glioma (brain tumors) to 229 controls. Cases were significantly less likely than controls to report a history of chickenpox (odds ratio, OR = 0.59). They also had significantly lower antibody levels to the varicella-zoster virus (OR = 0.41).

313.

Canniff J, Donson AM, et al. **Cytotoxicity of glioblastoma cells mediated ex vivo by varicella-zoster virus-specific T cells.** *J Neurovirol* 2011 Oct; 17(5): 448-54.

"Clinical or laboratory evidence of varicella-zoster virus infection has been consistently associated with lower glioma risk in case-control studies, suggesting a protective effect against glioma."

314.

Lee ST, Bracci P, et al. **Interaction of allergy history and antibodies to specific varicella-zoster virus proteins on glioma risk.** *Int J Cancer* 2014 May 1; 134(9): 2199-210.

"Glioma is the most common cancer of the central nervous system but with few confirmed risk factors. It has been inversely associated with chickenpox, shingles and seroreactivity to varicella virus."

315.

Childhood diseases experienced early in life protect against many different types of cancer later in life

"The results of this study consistently show a lower cancer risk in patients with a history of febrile infectious childhood diseases."

Albonico HU, Bräker HU, Hüsler J. **Febrile infectious childhood diseases in the history of cancer patients and matched controls.** *Med Hypotheses* 1998 Oct; 51(4): 315-20.

- Scientists compared 379 cancer patients with 379 controls to determine whether febrile infectious childhood diseases are associated with a reduced risk of cancer in adulthood.

- Adults were significantly protected against non-breast cancers — genital, prostate, gastrointestinal, skin, lung, ear-nose-throat, and others — if they contracted measles (OR = 0.45), rubella (OR = 0.38) or chickenpox (OR = 0.62) earlier in life.

- The total number of febrile infectious childhood diseases was also associated with a significantly decreased risk of cancer. For example, there was a 20% reduction in the risk of cancer later in life for every case of measles, mumps, rubella, chickenpox, pertussis, or scarlet fever experienced earlier in life.

- Adults with a history of three or four febrile infections were 60% less likely to develop non-breast cancers than adults who never had a febrile infection (OR = 0.40). Those with more than four febrile infections were 76% less likely to develop non-breast cancers (OR = 0.24).

- There was no statistically significant association between febrile infectious childhood diseases and breast cancer.

316.

There is a correlation between modern health practices that reduced infectious disease rates and increased cancer rates

"With a decreasing mortality from infectious illnesses, there may have been a reduction in the activation of immunological mechanisms against transformed cells in early phases of carcinogenesis."

Mastrangelo G, Fadda E, Milan G. **Cancer increased after a reduction of infections in the first half of this century in Italy: etiologic and preventive implications.** *Eur J Epidemiol* 1998 Dec; 14(8): 749-54.

- This paper compared a large reduction of infections in the first half of the 20th century in Italy with an increased rate of cancers.
- Studies show that cancer cells may be destroyed by a person's immune response to infectious disease. Conversely, cancer growth may be due to fewer non-lethal exposures to germs.
- Every 2% decrease in mortality from infectious disease was followed by a 2% increase in cancer mortality ten years later.
- This paper provides strong evidence of an association between decreased rates of infectious diseases and increased rates of cancer.

317.

Hoffmann, FL. **The mortality from cancer in the western hemisphere.** *J Cancer Res* January 1916 1; 21.

- This paper analyzed mortality rates in four large American cities during the late 19th and early 20th centuries.
- During this period, modern health practices dramatically reduced cases of smallpox, diphtheria and other infectious diseases. However, following this decline, the cancer death rate increased by 55%.

318.

Numerous studies confirm that acute infectious diseases protect against several types of cancer

"Many new vaccines have been introduced in recent years to counter common, and some less common, infectious diseases. The higher incidence of some cancers amongst individuals of a higher socio-economic status may reflect the negative aspects of reduced exposure to acute infections."

Hoption Cann SA, van Netten JP, et al. **Acute infections as a means of cancer prevention: opposing effects to chronic infections?** *Cancer Detect Prev* 2006; 30(1): 83-93.

- This paper examined the historical literature and epidemiological evidence (case control and cohort studies) on the relationship between acute infections and cancer.
- Several studies provide strong evidence that the increasing incidence of cancer in the early 20th century was due to the decreasing incidence of acute infectious diseases.
- Children who are exposed to febrile infectious diseases gain significant protection against multiple cancers in adulthood.
- Adults who were exposed to common acute infections derive significant protection against brain tumors, melanoma, and multiple cancers.
- A higher frequency of infections correlates with a greater protective effect against cancer.
- Infections accompanied by a fever — febrile infections — give the best protection against cancer. Fever suppression during infection may significantly increase morbidity and mortality.
- Although acute infections are protective against cancer, some chronic infections can lead to malignancies.

319.

Measles and other childhood infections protect against cancer of the lymph system

"Our findings provide additional support to the hypothesis that infections by most common childhood pathogens may protect against Hodgkin lymphoma.... In addition, our study shows that measles may provide a protective effect against non-Hodgkin lymphoma."

Montella M, Maso LD, et al. **Do childhood diseases affect NHL and HL risk? A case-control study from northern and southern Italy.** *Leuk Res* 2006 Aug; 30(8): 917-22.

- Scientists compared 225 people with non-Hodgkin lymphoma and 62 people with Hodgkin lymphoma to 504 people without cancer of the lymph system.

- This paper provides evidence that contracting measles in childhood reduces the risk of developing lymphatic cancer in adulthood.

320.

Alexander FE, Jarrett RF, et al. **Risk factors for Hodgkin's disease by Epstein-Barr virus (EBV) status: prior infection by EBV and other agents.** *Br J Cancer* 2000 Mar; 82(5): 1117-21.

"These results support previous evidence that early exposure to infection protects against Hodgkin's disease."

- Scientists compared 118 young adults (16-24 years of age) diagnosed with Hodgkin's disease to 237 gender- and age-matched controls.

- Infection with measles during childhood was significantly protective against developing Hodgkin's disease (OR = 0.53).

- Infection with two or more childhood diseases (measles, mumps, rubella, chickenpox or pertussis) was significantly protective against developing Hodgkin's disease (OR = 0.45).

321.

Lymph cancer is more likely in adults who were not infected with measles, mumps, or rubella during childhood

"Our population-based data...showed some evidence that childhood infections delayed to an older age increased risk of Epstein-Barr virus-positive Hodgkin's lymphoma in young adults."

Glaser SL, Keegan TH, et al. **Exposure to childhood infections and risk of Epstein-Barr virus-defined Hodgkin's lymphoma in women.** *Int J Cancer* 2005 Jul 1; 115(4): 599-605.

- Hodgkin's lymphoma (or Hodgkin's disease) is a cancer of lymph tissue, which is found in the lymph nodes, spleen, liver and bone marrow.

- Epstein-Barr virus (EBV) is found in some lymph tumors. (Infectious mononucleosis is delayed EBV infection.)

- This study was designed to investigate whether common childhood infections influence the risk of developing Hodgkin's lymphoma, and whether the risk varies when EBV is detected in lymph tumors.

- Scientists compared 268 women diagnosed with Hodgkin's lymphoma to 325 gender- and age-matched controls without the disease.

- Having at least one of three common childhood illnesses (measles, mumps or rubella) reduced the risk of EBV-positive Hodgkin's lymphoma in women 19 to 44 years of age (OR = 0.30).

- Having a history of measles before age 10 versus after age 10 (delayed) provided significant protection against EBV-positive Hodgkin's lymphoma (OR = 0.04).

322.

Hodgkin's disease is more likely in adults who were not infected with pertussis, measles, mumps, chickenpox or influenza during childhood

"Risk ratios of Hodgkin's disease tended to be lower for men who had experienced various common contagious diseases in childhood."

Paffenbarger RS Jr, Wing AL, Hyde RT. **Characteristics in youth indicative of adult-onset Hodgkin's disease.** *J Natl Cancer Inst* 1977 May; 58(5): 1489-91.

- This study compared 45 men who died of Hodgkin's disease to 180 controls.
- Men who died of Hodgkin's disease had fewer common contagious diseases in childhood than controls.
- A history of pertussis, measles, mumps, chickenpox, or influenza reduced the risk of dying from Hodgkin's disease.

323.

Gutensohn N, Cole P. **Childhood social environment and Hodgkin's disease.** *N Engl J Med* 1981; 304: 135-40.

"Risk (of Hodgkin's disease) is associated with a set of factors that tend to decrease or delay early exposure to infections."

- This study compared 225 people with Hodgkin's disease to 447 controls.
- Individuals with five or more siblings had nearly half the risk of Hodgkin's disease compared to those who had only one or none. The risk was also reduced in persons of a late birth order.
- Individuals with Hodgkin's disease were twice as likely to have lived in single family homes rather than multiple-family homes and had fewer playmates than controls during childhood.

324.

Early exposure to common infections develops and matures the immune system, significantly reducing the risk of lymph cancer

"Early exposure to other children at nursery school and daycare seems to decrease the risk of Hodgkin's lymphoma in young adults, most likely by facilitating childhood exposure to common infections and promoting maturation of cellular immunity."

Chang ET, Zheng T, et al. **Childhood social environment and Hodgkin's lymphoma: new findings from a population-based case-control study.** *Cancer Epidemiol Biomarkers Prev* 2004 Aug; 13(8): 1361-70.

- This study compared 565 people with Hodgkin's lymphoma to 679 controls.
- People 15 to 54 years of age who attended nursery school or daycare for at least one year during early childhood had a significantly reduced risk of developing Hodgkin's lymphoma (OR = 0.64).

325.

Rudant J, Orsi L, et al. **Childhood Hodgkin's lymphoma, non-Hodgkin's lymphoma and factors related to the immune system: the Escale Study (SFCE).** *Int J Cancer* 2011 Nov 1; 129(9): 2236-47.

"An abnormal maturation of the immune system may play a role in childhood Hodgkin's lymphoma or non-Hodgkin's lymphoma."

- This study compared 128 children with Hodgkin's lymphoma and 164 children with non-Hodgkin's lymphoma to 1,312 children without cancer of the lymph system.
- Children with cancer of the lymph system were significantly less likely than controls to have had common infections in early childhood (OR = 0.30). They were also less likely to have attended daycare or to have had two or more older siblings, conditions that are proxies for exposure to infections.

326.

Early exposure to infectious disease significantly reduces the risk of childhood leukemia

"This analysis provides strong support for an association between exposure to common infections in early childhood and a reduced risk of acute lymphoblastic leukemia."

Urayama KY, Buffler PA, et al. **A meta-analysis of the association between day-care attendance and childhood acute lymphoblastic leukaemia.** *Int J Epidemiol* 2010 Jun; 39(3): 718-32.

- This paper analyzed 14 studies, including 6,108 cases, to determine whether early exposure to infection is protective against acute lymphoblastic leukemia.
- Daycare attendance and social activity were proxies for exposure to infection.
- The combined result of the 14 studies confirms that exposure to infection in early childhood, as measured by daycare attendance and/or social activity, is associated with a significant reduction in the risk of developing acute lymphoblastic leukemia (OR = 0.76).

327.

van Steensel-Moll HA, Valkenburg HA, et al. **Childhood leukemia and infectious diseases in the first year of life: a register-based case-control study.** *Am J Epidemiol* 1986 Oct; 124(4): 590-94.

- This study investigated whether infectious diseases in the first year of life are associated with acute lymphocytic leukemia.
- In the Netherlands, scientists accessed a nationwide register of children with leukemia and compared them with gender- and age-matched controls.
- Infants who contracted primary childhood infections had a 20% reduction in the risk of childhood leukemia. Infants who had serious infectious diseases (requiring hospitalization) had a 40% reduction in the risk of leukemia.

328.

Infants with the least exposure to common infections have the greatest risk of developing childhood leukemia

"These results support the hypothesis that reduced exposure to infection in the first few months of life increases the risk of developing acute lymphoblastic leukemia. We conclude that some degree of early exposure to infection seems to be important for child health."

Gilham C, Peto J, et al. **Day care in infancy and risk of childhood acute lymphoblastic leukaemia: findings from UK case-control study**. *BMJ* 2005 June 2; 330: 1294.

- Scientists compared 1,286 British children with acute lymphoblastic leukemia to 6,305 children without cancer. Social activity and daycare during infancy were used as proxies for early exposure to infections.
- Infants with informal daycare outside the home were significantly protected against acute lymphoblastic leukemia (OR = 0.62). Infants who attended formal daycare at least twice a week (with at least four children) had a 52% reduced risk of developing acute lymphoblastic leukemia (OR = 0.48).
- Infants who started daycare in the first 3 months of life had greater reductions in risk than infants who started daycare after the first 3 months of life.

329.

Jourdan-Da Silva N, Perel Y, et al. **Infectious diseases in the first year of life, perinatal characteristics and childhood acute leukaemia.** *Br J Cancer* 2004 Jan 12; 90(1): 139-45.

"This study supports the hypothesis that early common infections may play a protective role in the etiology of childhood leukemia."

- This study compared 473 French children with acute leukemia to 567 controls. Infants who attended daycare starting before 3 months of age had a significantly reduced risk of developing acute leukemia (OR = 0.60).

330.

Early exposure to infections is protective against leukemia

"Evidence from a growing number of studies indicates that exposure to common infections early in life may be protective against childhood acute lymphoblastic leukemia."

Urayama KY, Ma X, et al. **Early life exposure to infections and risk of childhood acute lymphoblastic leukemia.** *Int J Cancer* 2011 Apr 1; 128(7): 1632-43.

- This study compared 669 children with acute lymphoblastic leukemia (ALL) and 977 controls to assess potential risk factors.
- Non-Hispanic white children had a reduced risk of ALL if they attended daycare by the age of 6 months (OR = 0.90) or had an older sibling (OR = 0.68). Both of these conditions are proxies for exposure to infections.
- In Hispanic children with ear infections before 6 months of age, there was a significant protective effect against ALL (OR = 0.45).

331.

Petridou E, Kassimos D, et al. **Age of exposure to infections and risk of childhood leukaemia.** *BMJ* 1993 Sep 25; 307: 774.

"Our results are compatible with previous suggestions in indicating that early attendance at creches reduces the risk of childhood leukemia, presumably by reducing the age of exposure to infectious agents."

- This study compared 136 Greek children diagnosed with leukemia and 187 controls to assess potential risk factors.
- Children who attended a creche (nursery) for at least 3 months in the first 2 years of life were significantly protected against childhood leukemia (relative risk, RR = 0.28). (Attendance at creches where children are crowded together enables effective transmission of infectious agents.)

332.

MMR, DPT and hepatitis B vaccination increase the risk of childhood leukemia

Buckley JD, Buckley CM, et al. **Epidemiological characteristics of childhood acute lymphocytic leukemia. Analysis by immunophenotype. The Children's Cancer Group.** *Leukemia* 1994 May; 8(5): 856-64.

- This study compared 990 children with acute lymphocytic leukemia to 1,636 cancer controls, and 404 cases matched to 440 community controls.
- Children who received MMR (measles, mumps, rubella) vaccination had a significantly elevated risk of acute lymphocytic leukemia (OR = 1.7).

333.

Innis MD. **Immunisation and childhood leukaemia.** *Lancet* 1965 Mar 13; 1(7385): 605.

- This study compared 59 children hospitalized with leukemia to a control group of 343 children without leukemia.
- Children who received DPT (diphtheria, pertussis, tetanus) vaccination had a significantly elevated risk of leukemia.

334.

Ma X, Does M, et al. **Hepatitis B vaccination and the risk of childhood leukemia**. Presented at the 93rd Annual Conference of the American Association for Cancer Research, 2002, San Francisco, CA, USA.

- The authors of this (unpublished) paper compared 167 children with leukemia to matched controls. Data was accessed from the Northern California Childhood Leukemia Study (NCCLS).
- Children who received 3 or more doses of hepatitis B vaccines had a significantly increased risk of leukemia (OR = 2.6). Infants who received hepatitis B vaccines were approximately 5 times more likely to develop leukemia.

335.

Measles infections can reverse cancer; the measles virus may be used as a treatment against human cancers

"This study demonstrates the efficacy of the measles virus against human melanoma."

Donnelly OG, Errington-Mais F, et al. **Measles virus causes immunogenic cell death in human melanoma.** *Gene Ther* 2013 Jan; 20(1): 7-15.

- Measles infections have been known to cause spontaneous cancer remissions.
- This study shows how the measles virus magnifies anti-tumor activity and provides evidence of its potential as a treatment against human melanoma.

336.

Touchefeu Y, Schick U, Harrington KJ. **Measles virus: a future therapeutic agent in oncology?** *Med Sci (Paris)* 2012 Apr; 28(4): 388-94.

- Tumor regressions have occurred after measles infection. This paper reviews the therapeutic use of attenuated strains of measles to kill cancer cells.

337.

Russell SJ, Peng KW. **Measles virus for cancer therapy.** *Curr Top Microbiol Immunol* 2009; 330: 213-41.

"Oncolytic (cancer destroying) viruses hold considerable promise as novel therapeutic agents for the treatment of human malignancies."

- Attenuated measles viruses can be engineered to enhance their naturally occurring anti-cancer properties and target specific tumors.
- Measles viruses are currently being tested to treat ovarian cancer, brain tumors and cancer of the bone marrow.

338.

Measles, mumps and chickenpox viruses have cancer-destroying properties

"Tumor-bearing mice treated with one thousand times the vaccine dose of each of the three [measles and mumps] viruses responded favorably to therapy with significant prolongations in survival."

Myers R, Greiner S, et al. **Oncolytic activities of approved mumps and measles vaccines for therapy of ovarian cancer.** *Cancer Gene Ther* 2005 Jul; 12(7): 593-99.

- In this study, scientists sought to measure the oncolytic (cancer destroying) properties of two measles viruses and one mumps virus by treating tumor-bearing mice with high concentrations of these viruses.
- The measles and mumps viruses killed malignant tumor cells allowing the treated mice to live longer than untreated mice.
- This study supports data showing the anti-cancer benefits of previously common childhood diseases, measles and mumps.

339.

Leske H, Haase R, et al. **Varicella zoster virus infection of malignant glioma cell cultures: a new candidate for oncolytic virotherapy?** *Anticancer Res* 2012 Apr; 32(4): 1137-44.

"Varicella zoster virus exhibits an intrinsic oncolytic potential in malignant glioma cell cultures and might be a novel candidate for virotherapy in glioblastoma multiforme."

- Glioblastoma multiforme is the most common and highly aggressive type of brain tumor.
- This study investigated the cancer-destroying potential of the varicella-zoster virus in malignant glioma cell cultures. Rapid destruction of the tumor cells occurred in vitro.

Vitamin A and Measles

Measles can be a dangerous disease, especially in third world nations where children are malnourished. In developed nations, measles can be severe when it infects people living in impoverished communities with poor nutrition, sanitation and inadequate health care. Complications are also more likely when the disease strikes infants, adults, and anyone with a compromised immune system.

Several studies show that severe cases of measles in children are associated with vitamin A deficiency. When patients with measles are given high doses of vitamin A, their complication rates and chances of dying are significantly reduced. The World Health Organization and American Academy of Pediatrics recommend administering 200,000 international units (IU) of vitamin A to children older than 1 year of age to be given immediately when measles is diagnosed, with a second dose given the following day. Infants who are 6-12 months of age should be given 2 doses of 100,000 IU of vitamin A. Infants who are younger than 6 months of age should be given 2 doses of 50,000 IU of vitamin A.

340.

Vitamin A supplementation is highly protective against complications and death from measles

"Vitamin A deficiency may be a large factor in determining outcome of measles in Africa, just as it seems to affect morbidity and mortality in Asia. When a child with marginal stores [of vitamin A] gets measles, the available vitamin A is quickly depleted, presumably reducing the ability to resist secondary infections or their consequences. This would exacerbate the already reduced immunocompetence thought to be associated with measles infection."

Barclay AJ, Foster A, Sommer A. **Vitamin A supplements and mortality related to measles: a randomised clinical trial.** *BMJ* 1987 Jan 31; 294: 294-96.

- African children with measles were divided into two groups. The first group received routine treatment. The second group received the same treatment plus 200,000 IU (international units) of vitamin A on hospital admission and again the next day.

- The death rate in children under 2 years of age declined by 87% in the group that received vitamin A supplementation (2.2% mortality) when compared to the group that only received routine treatment (16.7% mortality).

- The death rate in all children who received the routine treatment plus vitamin A supplementation was nearly half that of the children who received routine treatment alone — 6.8% compared to 13%.

- The death rate in extremely malnourished children was many times higher than that of better nourished children. However, vitamin A was protective against complications from measles and lowered mortality regardless of the child's nutritional status.

341.

The World Health Organization (WHO) recommends high doses of vitamin A for children with measles to reduce their risk of complications and death

"Immediate vitamin A therapy significantly reduces the risk of excessive measles case fatality. It is therefore recommended to treat children with high-dose vitamin A supplements during episodes of measles."

WHO/UNICEF/IVAGG Task Force. **Vitamin A Supplements — A Guide to Their Use in The Treatment and Prevention of Vitamin A Deficiency and Xerophthalmia (second edition).** Geneva: WHO, 1997: 8.

- The World Health Organization (WHO) and American Academy of Pediatrics recommend administering 200,000 IU of vitamin A to children older than 1 year of age, (if vitamin A deficiency may be present) to be given immediately upon a measles diagnosis, with a second dose given the following day.

- Infants who are 6-12 months of age should be given 2 doses of 100,000 IU of vitamin A. Infants who are younger than 6 months of age should be given 2 doses of 50,000 IU of vitamin A.

342.

Sudfeld CR, Navar AM, et al. **Effectiveness of measles vaccination and vitamin A treatment.** *Int J Epidemiol* 2010 Apr; 39 Suppl 1: i48-55.

"The World Health Organization (WHO) recommends vitamin A treatment of measles consisting of two doses of 50,000 IU for infants under 6 months of age, 100,000 IU for those 6 months to 1 year of age, and 200,000 IU for individuals over one year of age."

- Vitamin A treatment for measles recommended by WHO was found to reduce measles mortality by 62% (relative risk, RR = 0.38).

343.

Vitamin A supplementation for children with measles, as recommended by the World Health Organization (WHO), is effective at saving lives

"We conclude that 200,000 IU of vitamin A repeated on 2 days should be used for the treatment of measles as recommended by the World Health Organization in children admitted to hospitals in areas where the case fatality is high."

D'Souza RM, D'Souza R. **Vitamin A for the treatment of children with measles — a systematic review.** *J Trop Pediatr* 2002 Dec; 48(6): 323-27.

- Severe cases of measles are associated with a deficiency of vitamin A.
- High doses of vitamin A — 200,000 IU given for 2 days to hospitalized children with measles — significantly reduced overall mortality by 64% and pneumonia-specific mortality by 67%. Mortality was reduced by 83% in children under 2 years of age (RR = 0.17).

344.

Coutsoudis A, Broughton M, et al. **Vitamin A supplementation reduces measles morbidity in young African children: a randomized, placebo-controlled, double-blind trial.** *Am J Clin Nutr* 1991 Nov; 54(5): 890-95.

"[This study] supports the current World Health Organization recommendations for vitamin A supplementation during measles."

- African children 4 months to 2 years of age hospitalized with severe measles were divided into two groups and either received a World Health Organization (WHO) recommended treatment of vitamin A or placebo.
- The morbidity (severity) of the disease was reduced by more than 80% in the group that received vitamin A supplementation. The improvement in health was mainly due to reduced respiratory tract infection.

345.

Studies provide evidence that vitamin A protects children against complications and death from measles

"Using two doses of vitamin A (200,000 IU) on consecutive days was associated with a reduction in the risk of mortality in children under the age of two years and a reduction in the risk of pneumonia-specific mortality."

Huiming Y, Chaomin W, Meng M. **Vitamin A for treating measles in children.** *Cochrane Database Syst Rev* 2005 Oct 19; (4): CD001479.

- This paper analyzed several studies to determine whether high-dose vitamin A supplementation for children, initiated after measles is diagnosed, prevents mortality, pneumonia, and other complications of the disease.
- Vitamin A therapy for children under 2 years of age with measles significantly reduces their risk of succumbing to complications of the disease and dying.

346.

Hussey GD, Klein M. **A randomized, controlled trial of vitamin A in children with severe measles.** *N Engl J Med* 1990 Jul 19; 323(3): 160-64.

"For the group treated with vitamin A, risk of death or a major complication during the hospital stay was half that of the control group."

- Children hospitalized with measles were randomly divided into two groups. One group received the usual treatment plus an oral dose of 400,000 IU of vitamin A. The other group received the usual treatment plus a placebo.
- Compared with the placebo group, the children who were treated with vitamin A recovered more quickly from pneumonia and diarrhea, had less croup, and spent fewer days hospitalized.
- Ten of the 12 children who died were in the control group that did not receive vitamin A supplementation.

347.

Vitamin A treatment for children with measles increases their antibody levels, protecting them from severe complications

"Our data show that many children younger than 2 years in New York City have low vitamin A levels when ill with measles, and that such children seem to have lower measles-specific antibody levels and increased morbidity. Clinicians may wish to consider vitamin A therapy for children younger than 2 years with severe measles."

Frieden TR, Sowell AL, et al. **Vitamin A levels and severity of measles. New York City.** *Am J Dis Child* 1992 Feb; 146(2): 182-86.

- Vitamin A levels in children younger than 2 years of age, with measles, were measured.
- Children with low vitamin A levels were more likely to be hospitalized and to have a higher fever (at least 104° F) that lasted for 7 days or longer.
- Children with low vitamin A levels had fewer antibodies against measles.

348.

Coutsoudis A, Kiepiela P, et al. **Vitamin A supplementation enhances specific IgG antibody levels and total lymphocyte numbers while improving morbidity in measles.** *Pediatr Infect Dis J* 1992 Mar;11(3): 203-9.

- Children who were hospitalized with measles and supplemented with vitamin A showed an increase in total number of lymphocytes and measles IgG antibodies, which have been shown to correlate with an improved outcome in measles.
- The children who received vitamin A treatment for measles had significant reductions in the severity of their disease when compared to children who did not receive vitamin A supplementation.

349.

Older children with measles, and babies of breastfeeding mothers, may benefit from high-dose vitamin A supplementation

"We conclude that a policy of high dose oral vitamin A (400,000 IU) supplementation in measles provides benefits which are equivalent to those previously observed only in controlled research trials, that it is highly cost effective, and that it should form part of the routine case management of all children hospitalized with measles."

Hussey GD , Klein M. **Routine high-dose vitamin A therapy for children hospitalized with measles.** *J Trop Pediatr* 1993 Dec; 39(6): 342-45.

- This study analyzed the records of 1,720 children less than 15 years of age who were hospitalized for measles. Some of the children received high-dose vitamin A therapy; the remaining children received standard therapy.
- When compared to the group of children on standard therapy, children who received high-dose vitamin A therapy spent less time in the hospital, had a reduced need for intensive care, and a lower death rate (1.6% versus 5%).

350.

Sommer A. **Vitamin A prophylaxis**. *Arch Dis Child* 1997; 77: 191-94. [Annotation.]

"Prompt administration of large doses of vitamin A to children with moderate to severe measles, particularly if they may be vitamin A deficient, can reduce individual mortality by 50% and prevent or moderate the severity of complications."

- Children aged 6 months to 6 years who contract measles can be treated with 200,000 IU of vitamin A, two days in a row, to dramatically reduce complications and death from the disease.
- Women who have recently given birth are advised to receive 200,000 IU of vitamin A to increase the amount transferred in breast milk to the baby.

351.

Newborn boys and adults with measles gain protection from high-dose vitamin A supplementation

"Vitamin A supplementation compared with placebo tended to be associated with less measles hospitalization or death during the first 6 months of life in boys, but not in girls."

Diness BR, Martins CL, et al. **The effect of high-dose vitamin A supplementation at birth on measles incidence during the first 12 months of life in boys and girls: an unplanned study within a randomised trial.** *Br J Nutr* 2011 Jun; 105(12): 1819-22.

- This study sought to determine whether vitamin A supplementation (50,000 IU) given to newborns with normal birth weight would reduce their risk of hospitalization or death during a measles epidemic.
- Vitamin A supplementation at birth was beneficial for males but not for females.

352.

Melenotte C, Brouqui P, Botelho-Nevers E. **Severe measles, vitamin A deficiency, and the Roma community in Europe.** *Emerg Infect Dis* 2012 Sep; 18(9): 1537-39. [Letter.]

"We conclude that all adults who have measles should be assessed for vitamin A and retinol-binding protein levels and should be considered for vitamin A supplementation, as are children."

- Studies have shown that severe cases of measles in children are associated with vitamin A deficiency.
- This paper confirms that severe cases of measles in adults are associated with malnutrition and low levels of vitamin A.

353.

Evidence that vitamins A and D protect children against complications and death from measles has been available since 1932

"The use of a concentrate rich in vitamin A as a prophylactic against secondary infections in a population of young children known to have been exposed to measles might well repay further study."

Ellison JB. **Intensive vitamin therapy in measles.** *Br Med J* 1932 Oct 15; 2(3745): 708-11.

- Between October 1931 and April 1932, 600 children under 5 years of age who were hospitalized for measles were divided into two equal groups. One group received "a rich concentrate of vitamins A and D" daily for 1-3 weeks, starting on the day of admission. The other group received normal treatment.

- The hospitalized children who received the vitamin A and D supplements were significantly less likely to die compared to the children who did not receive the vitamin therapy (3.7% versus 8.7%).

- Pulmonary complications were less severe in the vitamin-treated group than in the control group.

Vitamin D and Influenza

Ultraviolet radiation from the sun induces vitamin D production in the skin. Sufficient vitamin D is essential to a healthy immune system. In winter, solar radiation is weak, causing widespread vitamin D deficiency. In regions of the world with higher latitudes and lower amounts of ultraviolet radiation, influenza epidemics peak around the winter solstice and end in the sunny months. Thus, influenza infection may be a sign of vitamin D deficiency.

In developed nations, about 40% of pregnant women and half of all newborns and infants have insufficient vitamin D. A high percentage of children and adults have insufficient vitamin D as well. Low vitamin D levels in pregnant women have been linked to several diseases in their babies, including infant wheezing and respiratory infections. Children and adults with insufficient vitamin D are at risk to develop influenza and other respiratory infections. Middle-aged and older adults with low vitamin D levels are significantly more likely to die from any cause when compared to adults with higher vitamin D levels.

The studies in this chapter provide strong evidence that vitamin D supplementation significantly reduces the risk of influenza, pneumonia and other respiratory infections. Vitamin D supplementation is recommended for pregnant women, infants, children and adults. Some doctors also recommend vitamin D supplementation for healthcare workers who may be hesitant to take a vaccine.

The common assumption that influenza is caused by different viral strains every year rather than influenced by host immunity may need to be reconsidered. Viral strains might only manifest as disease under particular conditions related to a weakening of the host immune system. The concept of herd immunity may need to be redefined to include innate immunity achieved when a percentage of the population acquires adequate vitamin D levels to exert immune pressure on the circulating influenza virus.

354.

Vitamin D is protective against acute respiratory tract infections, including influenza

"The data in this study suggests that supplementing with vitamin D to raise the concentrations in the general population to above 38 ng/mL could result in a significant health benefit by reducing the burden of illness from viral infections."

Sabetta JR, DePetrillo P, et al. **Serum 25-hydroxyvitamin D and the incidence of acute viral respiratory tract infections in healthy adults.** *PLoS One* 2010 June 14; 5(6): e11088.

- Viral respiratory tract infections have seasonal variations. For example, influenza epidemics do not occur in the summer, even when the virus is freely circulating and crowds of people gather together.

- Influenza epidemics happen simultaneously in the fall and winter at the same temperate latitudes throughout the planet.

- This study was conducted to determine if serum vitamin D levels in healthy adults are related to acute viral respiratory tract infections, including influenza.

- Serum 25-hydroxyvitamin D concentrations in 198 healthy adults were measured monthly during the fall and winter of 2009-2010. Acute viral infections were diagnosed in 84 patients during the study.

- A vitamin D concentration of 38 ng/mL (nanograms per milliliter) or higher significantly reduced by half the risk of developing an acute viral respiratory tract infection.

- The incidence of infection was 2.7 times lower and the percentage of days ill was 4.9 times lower in the group that maintained vitamin D levels of 38 ng/mL or higher during the entire study period as compared to the group with levels below 38 ng/mL.

- There were no differences among those who took supplements, vitamins (other than vitamin D), herbs, or influenza vaccines.

355.

Eleven randomized studies show that vitamin D significantly reduces the risk of influenza, pneumonia and other respiratory infections

"Our meta-analysis of randomized controlled trials indicates a protective effect of vitamin D supplementation against respiratory tract infections."

Bergman P, Lindh AU, et al. **Vitamin D and respiratory tract infections: a systematic review and meta-analysis of randomized controlled trials.** *PLoS ONE* 2013, 8(6): e65835.

- Researchers conducted a systematic review and meta-analysis of all placebo-controlled studies assessing the effect of vitamin D supplementation on respiratory tract infections such as influenza and *Streptococcus pneumoniae*.

- Eleven studies with 5,660 participants (6 months to 75 years of age) met the inclusion criteria.

- The combined results of the 11 randomized placebo-controlled studies showed that oral vitamin D supplementation significantly reduces the risk of both upper and lower respiratory tract infections (OR = 0.64).

- The protective benefits of vitamin D were even greater in studies using more frequent but smaller (daily) doses rather than less frequent but larger (bolus) doses (OR = 0.51 versus OR = 0.86).

- The age of the study participants did not affect the results.

356.

Vitamin D significantly protects adults and children against influenza, pneumonia, and other respiratory infections

"According to this systematic review and meta-analysis, vitamin D significantly reduces respiratory tract infection related events as compared to placebo. Beneficial effect of vitamin D was observed in children as well as adults. On the basis of this study, we can conclude that vitamin D is useful in prevention of respiratory tract infections."

Charan J, Goyal JP, et al. **Vitamin D for prevention of respiratory tract infections: A systematic review and meta-analysis.** *J Pharmacol Pharmacother* 2012 Oct-Dec; 3(4): 300-303.

- This paper analyzed five randomized placebo-controlled clinical studies that investigated whether vitamin D supplementation can prevent respiratory tract infections such as influenza, pneumonia, and the common cold.

- Vitamin D supplementation significantly reduced the number of respiratory tract infections in adults (odds ratio, OR = 0.65) and children (OR = 0.58) when compared to groups that did not receive supplementation.

357.

Borella E, Nesher G, et al. **Vitamin D: a new anti-infective agent?** *Ann NY Acad Sci* 2014 May; 1317: 76-83.

"Vitamin D may be acting as a panacean antibiotic agent and thus may be useful as an adjuvant therapy in diverse infections."

- Low vitamin D levels are associated with influenza, pneumonia, and upper respiratory infections.

358.

Vitamin D supplementation significantly protects school children against influenza and asthma attacks

"This study suggests that vitamin D_3 supplementation during the winter may reduce the incidence of influenza A, especially in specific subgroups of schoolchildren."

Urashima M, Segawa T, et al. **Randomized trial of vitamin D supplementation to prevent seasonal influenza A in schoolchildren.** *Am J Clin Nutr* 2010; 91: 1255-60.

- This randomized, double-blind, placebo-controlled study investigated the effect of vitamin D_3 supplements — 1200 IU daily through winter — on the incidence of seasonal influenza A in school children.

- Influenza A occurred in 10.8% of children in the vitamin D_3 group compared with 18.6% of children in the placebo group — a significant 42% reduction (relative risk, RR = 0.58).

- Vitamin D_3 significantly reduced the incidence of influenza A within 60 days.

- In children with a previous diagnosis of asthma, vitamin D_3 supplementation significantly suppressed asthma attacks (RR = 0.17).

359.

Vitamin D supplementation protects black women against colds and influenza

"These reports provide a rationale for vitamin D supplementation in the prevention of colds and influenza. Since there is an epidemic of vitamin D insufficiency in the United States, the public health impact of this observation could be great."

Aloia JF, Li-Ng M. **Re: epidemic influenza and vitamin D.** *Epidemiol Infect* 2007 Oct; 135(7): 1095-96; author reply 1097-98. [Letter.]

- This 3-year randomized controlled trial was designed to study rates of bone loss, colds and influenza in postmenopausal black women.

- The women were divided into two groups. One group of 104 women were supplemented with 800 to 2000 IU of vitamin D_3 daily; the second group of 104 women received a placebo.

- Just 7.7% of women in the vitamin D group reported respiratory tract symptoms compared to 25% of women in the control group.

- Although colds and influenza mainly occur during the winter season when vitamin D produced from the sun is meager, women in the vitamin D group not only reported fewer respiratory infections, but when they did get sick, it was equally likely to occur at any time of the year, not just in the winter.

- Vitamin D supplementation ended the seasonality of colds and influenza.

360.

Cities with the least solar radiation and vitamin D had the worst death rates during the 1918-1919 influenza pandemic

"The potential role of vitamin D status in reducing secondary bacterial infections and loss of life in pandemic influenza requires further evaluation."

Grant WB, Giovannucci E. **The possible roles of solar ultraviolet-B radiation and vitamin D in reducing case-fatality rates from the 1918-1919 influenza pandemic in the United States.** *Dermatoendocrinol* 2009 Jul-Aug; 1(4): 215-19.

- Exposure to the sun — solar ultraviolet B radiation — induces biosynthesis of vitamin D, which has anti-microbial properties that may enhance immune defenses against influenza and secondary bacterial infections.

- This paper analyzed influenza and pneumonia death rates in 12 U.S. cities (of varying latitudes) during the 1918-1919 influenza pandemic to determine whether they were affected by solar ultraviolet-B radiation.

- U.S. cities closer to the equator (lower latitude) receive more solar ultraviolet-B radiation, a proxy for city-wide immune-enhancing vitamin D levels.

- There was an inverse relationship between ultraviolet B radiation and case-fatality rates of influenza (and pneumonia as a complication of influenza).

- During the 1918-1919 influenza pandemic, the lowest case-fatality rates tended to occur in cities with the lowest latitudes and highest quantities of solar ultraviolet B radiation, such as San Antonio, Texas.

- The highest influenza case-fatality rate was in New London, Connecticut, which had the highest latitude and least amount of ultraviolet B radiation of the 12 cities investigated.

- Fortifying food with higher amounts of vitamin D or providing vitamin D supplements should be considered as part of an overall preventive health program aimed at reducing influenza mortality rates.

361.

Influenza epidemics are due to weak winter sunlight, inducing vitamin D deficiency

"Without factoring in the effects of innate immunity, we must contort our logic to make sense of influenza's bewildering epidemiological contradictions."

Cannell JJ, Zasloff M, et al. **On the epidemiology of influenza.** *Virol J* 2008 Feb 25; 5:29.

- This paper critically examined 9 influenza perplexities. For example, Why is influenza seasonal? Where does the virus go between epidemics? Why do influenza epidemics occur simultaneously in countries of similar latitude?

- In winter, the sun's ultraviolet radiation is weak, causing vitamin D deficiency, concurrent impairments of innate immunity, and epidemics of influenza.

- Studies confirm that vitamin D offers protection against respiratory infections, including influenza.

362.

Cannell JJ, Vieth R, et al. **Epidemic influenza and vitamin D.** *Epidemiol Infect* 2006 Dec; 134(6): 1129-40.

- Ultraviolet radiation from the sun triggers vitamin D production in the skin. Vitamin D is essential to a healthy immune system.

- In winter, solar radiation is weak, causing widespread vitamin D deficiency. Influenza epidemics in temperate latitudes peak around the winter solstice and end in the sunny months — even though many potential victims lack antibodies against current strains of influenza.

- Influenza infection may be a sign of vitamin D deficiency.

- The concept of herd immunity may need to be redefined to include innate immunity achieved when a percentage of the population acquires adequate vitamin D levels to exert immune pressure on the circulating virus.

363.

Seasonal influenza occurs in the winter when solar radiation is weak and vitamin D levels are low

"The data support the hypothesis that high fluences of ultraviolet B radiation (vitamin D level), as occur in the summer, act in a protective manner with respect to influenza."

Juzeniene A, Ma LW, et al. **The seasonality of pandemic and non-pandemic influenzas: the roles of solar radiation and vitamin D.** *Int J Infect Dis* 2010 Dec; 14(12): e1099-1105.

- Seasonal variations in solar ultraviolet B radiation — higher in summer and lower in winter — cause seasonal variations in levels of vitamin D. This could affect immune responses to influenza.

- This paper studied pandemic and non-pandemic influenzas in five countries. Monthly influenza incidence and death rates were compared with monthly variations in ultraviolet B radiation.

- In temperate regions with higher latitudes and lower amounts of ultraviolet B radiation, virtually no vitamin D is produced in the skin during the winter when non-pandemic influenzas mostly occur.

- In tropical regions with year-round ultraviolet B radiation, there is virtually no seasonality of influenza.

- Low vitamin D levels may cause increased susceptibility to influenza.

364.

Influenza and pneumonia deaths primarily occur in the winter when solar radiation and vitamin D serum levels are low

"Our data are in agreement with the assumption that the high numbers of winter influenza and pneumonia deaths in Norway are related to low vitamin D levels in this season."

Moan J, Dahlback A, et al. **Influenza, solar radiation and vitamin D.** *Dermatoendocrinol* 2009 Nov; 1(6): 307-9.

- This paper studied influenza and pneumonia deaths in Norway from 1980-2000, comparing them with variations in ultraviolet B radiation and estimated vitamin D levels.

- Norway is located at 58 to 70 degrees latitude north. At just 25 degrees latitude north the rate of vitamin D synthesis in human skin is about five times greater in late June than in late December.

- Researchers found a strong seasonal variation. Nearly all of the influenza and pneumonia deaths in Norway occurred during the winter season when ultraviolet B radiation is weak and vitamin D photosynthesis and vitamin D serum levels are insufficient.

- Death rates for influenza and pneumonia are very low during the summer season when ultraviolet B radiation is strong and vitamin D status is best.

- This paper argues against the common assumption that influenza is caused by different viral strains every year rather than being host-related. Viral strains might only manifest as disease under particular conditions related to a weakening of the host immune system.

365.

Patients hospitalized with pneumonia are less likely to have a repeat episode or die if they have sufficient vitamin D

"A single high-dose oral vitamin D_3 supplementation to young children along with antibiotic treatment for pneumonia could reduce the occurrence of repeat episodes of pneumonia."

Manaseki-Holland S, Qader G, et al. **Effects of vitamin D supplementation to children diagnosed with pneumonia in Kabul: a randomised controlled trial.** *Trop Med Int Health* 2010 Oct; 15(10): 1148-55.

- In a double-blind randomized placebo-controlled study conducted in an Afghan hospital, 453 young children diagnosed with pneumonia were divided into two groups. One group received 100,000 IU of vitamin D_3 plus antibiotics. The other group received a placebo.

- Children who received vitamin D supplementation were less likely to have a repeat episode of pneumonia within 90 days (relative risk, RR = 0.78) and survived longer without having a repeat episode (hazard ratio, HR = 0.71) than children in the placebo group.

366.

Leow L, Simpson T, et al. **Vitamin D, innate immunity and outcomes in community acquired pneumonia.** *Respirology* 2011 May; 16(4): 611-16.

"25-hydroxyvitamin D deficiency is associated with increased mortality in patients admitted to hospital with community acquired pneumonia during winter."

- This study investigated an association between serum vitamin D levels and the risk of death in 112 patients admitted to a hospital with pneumonia.

- Pneumonia patients with a severe vitamin D deficiency (less than 30 nmol/L) were 12 times more likely to die within 30 days compared to patients with serum concentrations of vitamin D greater than 50 nmol/L (OR = 12.7).

367.

Insufficient serum vitamin D in pregnant women increases the risk of respiratory infections and wheezing in their babies

"In a population-based birth cohort with excellent 5-year follow-up, cord-blood 25-hydroxyvitamin D levels had significant inverse associations with the risk of respiratory infection and risk of childhood wheezing."

Camargo CA Jr, Ingham T, et al. **Cord-blood 25-hydroxyvitamin D levels and risk of respiratory infection, wheezing, and asthma.** *Pediatrics* 2011 Jan; 127(1): e180-87.

- The purpose of this study was to determine if serum vitamin D levels at birth correlate with the risk of respiratory infection during the first 3 months of life, and of wheezing and/or asthma throughout early childhood.

- Vitamin D levels were measured in the umbilical cord blood of 922 newborns.

- Newborns with vitamin D cord blood levels less than 25 nmol/L were twice as likely to develop a respiratory infection by 3 months of age compared to those with levels of 75 nmol/L or higher (OR = 2.04). They were also twice as likely to develop *any* type of infection by 3 months of age (OR = 2.36).

- Low vitamin D cord blood levels at birth significantly increased the risk of childhood wheezing by 15 months, 3 years, and 5 years of age (OR = 2.15).

- Every 10 nmol/L increase in the amount of vitamin D measured at birth decreased the cumulative risk of wheeze.

- Vitamin D levels in pregnant women might affect the developing fetal immune system and health of the newborn in the early months outside the womb.

368.

Vitamin D supplementation of pregnant women could decrease the risk of lower respiratory infections in their newborns

"Our findings suggest that newborns with subclinical vitamin D deficiency may have an increased risk of suffering from acute lower respiratory infection. The strong positive correlation between newborns' and mothers' 25-hydroxyvitamin D concentrations shows that adequate vitamin D supplementation of mothers should be emphasized during pregnancy especially in winter months."

Karatekin G, Kaya A, et al. **Association of subclinical vitamin D deficiency in newborns with acute lower respiratory infection and their mothers.** *Eur J Clin Nutr* 2009 Apr; 63(4): 473-77.

- The serum vitamin D levels of newborns with acute lower respiratory infection admitted to neonatal intensive care were compared to a control group of healthy newborns.
- The average vitamin D level of the hospitalized newborns (9.12 ng/mL) was significantly lower than those of the healthy newborns (16.33 ng/mL).
- The average vitamin D level in the mothers of the hospitalized newborns (13.38 ng/mL) was significantly lower than those of the mothers of the control group (22.79 ng/mL).
- The serum vitamin D levels of the newborns were highly correlated with their mothers' serum vitamin D levels.
- Vitamin D supplementation for pregnant women is recommended.

369.

Vitamin D reduces the risk of influenza and pneumonia in pregnant women, and protects infants from respiratory infections

"Pregnant women should be encouraged to increase their serum 25-hydroxyvitamin D levels to 40 to 80 ng/mL through supplementation with several thousand international units per day of vitamin D_3 or solar ultraviolet B when the sun is high enough that one's shadow is shorter than one's height."

Grant WB. **Pregnant women are at increased risk for severe A influenza because they have low serum 25-hydroxyvitamin D levels.** *Crit Care Med* 2010, 38(9): 1921. [Letter.]

- Vitamin D deficiency is common in pregnant women and in breastfed infants despite extensive use of prenatal vitamins (the doses are not high enough).

- Higher vitamin D levels will reduce the risk of influenza, pneumonia, viral infectious diseases, cancer, cardiovascular disease, autoimmune diseases, and complications of pregnancy. Supplementation is recommended.

370.

Grant CC, Kaur S, et al. **Reduced primary care respiratory infection visits following pregnancy and infancy vitamin D supplementation: a randomised controlled trial.** *Acta Paediatr* 2015 Apr; 104(4): 396-404.

"Vitamin D_3 supplementation during pregnancy and infancy reduces primary care visits for acute respiratory infection during early childhood."

- Scientists assigned 260 pregnant women and their infants to one of three groups to receive daily low doses of vitamin D, higher doses of vitamin D, or placebo.

- Children in the group that received higher doses of vitamin D had fewer acute respiratory infections from 6 to 18 months of age.

371.

Vitamin D deficiency in pregnant women and newborns significantly increases the risk of respiratory syncytial virus (RSV) infections during infancy

"Results of this prospective birth cohort study demonstrated that vitamin D deficiency is highly prevalent among healthy newborns in Western countries, and that neonates who are vitamin D deficient at birth have an increased risk of developing respiratory syncytial virus respiratory tract infections during infancy."

Belderbos ME, Houben ML, et al. **Cord blood vitamin D deficiency is associated with respiratory syncytial virus bronchiolitis.** *Pediatrics* 2011 Jun; 127(6): e1513-20.

- In developed nations, about 40% of pregnant women and half of all newborns and infants have insufficient vitamin D.

- Vitamin D deficiency in pregnant women has been linked to several diseases in their offspring, including type 1 diabetes, multiple sclerosis, schizophrenia, infant wheezing, and respiratory infections.

- This study was designed to determine whether low serum vitamin D levels in pregnant women and their newborns increase the risk of respiratory syncytial virus (RSV) infections.

- Vitamin D levels in the umbilical cord blood of 156 newborns were measured. Babies born with levels below 50 nmol/L were 6 times more likely than babies born with levels greater than 75 nmol/L to develop an RSV lower respiratory tract infection in the first year of life (relative risk, RR = 6.2).

- Vitamin D supplementation in pregnancy is strongly associated with cord blood concentrations in newborns. Low vitamin D in newborns is linked to a significantly increased risk of developing an RSV infection.

- Routine vitamin D supplementation during pregnancy could be an important way to prevent RSV infections during infancy.

372.

There is a statistically significant link between insufficient vitamin D and acute respiratory tract infections

"The findings from the present study contribute to the diversity of consequences already known to result from vitamin D insufficiency and recognized as carrying significant global public health implications."

Laaksi I, Ruohola JP, et al. **An association of serum vitamin D concentrations < 40 nmol/L with acute respiratory tract infection in young Finnish men.** *Am J Clin Nutr* 2007; 86: 714-17.

- This study sought to determine whether there is a link between low serum vitamin D levels and acute respiratory tract infections, such as pneumonia, bronchitis and sinusitis.

- The serum vitamin D levels of 756 young Finnish men serving on a military base were measured prior to a 6-month observational period during which physician-diagnosed respiratory tract infections were recorded, along with the number of days of absence from duty.

- Subjects with serum hydroxyvitamin D levels of less than 40 nmol/L (16 ng/mL) at the beginning of the 6-month observational period had significantly more days of absence from duty due to respiratory infections than did controls (incidence rate ratio, IRR = 1.63).

- Subjects who smoked had significantly lower serum vitamin D levels than controls. Subjects who exercised at least 5 hours per week before entering the military had significantly higher vitamin D levels compared to subjects who did not exercise prior to entering the military.

- This study provides strong evidence that vitamin D insufficiency significantly increases susceptibility to respiratory infections.

373.

Middle-aged and older adults with high levels of vitamin D are significantly less likely to die from respiratory disease and other causes

"This 13-year prospective study in a free-living, middle-aged and older British population provides additional support for the hypothesis that vitamin D status is associated with a range of important health outcomes including respiratory disease, cardiovascular disease, fractures, and total mortality. Highest mortality rates were observed in individuals with 25(OH)D concentrations below 30 nmol/L."

Khaw KT, Luben R, Wareham N. **Serum 25-hydroxyvitamin D, mortality, and incident cardiovascular disease, respiratory disease, cancers, and fractures: a 13-y prospective population study.** *Am J Clin Nutr* 2014 Nov; 100(5): 1361-70.

- 14,641 adults 42-82 years of age were placed into 5 groups based on their serum vitamin D levels: a) less than 30 nmol/L, b) 30 to < 50, c) 50 to < 70, d) 70 to < 90, and e) 90 or higher nmol/L. They were followed up for 13 years or until they died.

- The risk of dying from any cause was significantly lower in the adults with higher vitamin D levels. Adults with levels greater than 90 nmol/L were 34% less likely to die compared to those with less than 30 nmol/L (HR = 0.66).

- Adults with vitamin D levels greater than 90 nmol/L were 78% less likely to die from respiratory disease or respiratory infections compared to those with less than 30 nmol/L (HR = 0.22).

- Higher vitamin D levels were also shown to be significantly protective against cardiovascular disease and bone fractures.

- Vitamin D_3 was the predominant form of vitamin D.

- Raising vitamin D levels in the general population could provide significant health benefits without increasing risk.

374.

Insufficient vitamin D in children and adults is associated with respiratory infections; supplementation is recommended

"Vitamin D deficiency and insufficiency are common among school children in Xinxiang. Supplementation with food fortification or vitamin D for Chinese children is warranted."

Li PL, Tian YJ, et al. **The prevalence of vitamin D deficiency among schoolchildren: a cohort study from Xinxiang, China.** *J Pediatr Endocrinol Metab* 2015 May; 28(5-6): 629-33.

- There is an inverse relationship between vitamin D levels in children and number of respiratory infections.
- Serum vitamin D levels in 606 Chinese school children were measured; 47% of the children were deficient in vitamin D and 86% had insufficient levels. Vitamin D supplementation for children is recommended.

375.

Berry DJ, Hesketh K, et al. **Vitamin D status has a linear association with seasonal infections and lung function in British adults.** *Br J Nutr* 2011 Nov; 106(9): 1433-40.

"Vitamin D status had a linear relationship with respiratory infections and lung function."

- This study investigated the relationship between serum vitamin D levels, respiratory infections and lung function.
- Measurements of serum vitamin D levels, respiratory infections, and lung strength (forced expiration volume and forced vital capacity) on 6789 adults 45 years of age and older were collected and analyzed.
- Every 10 nmol/L increase in serum vitamin D levels significantly reduced the risk of respiratory infection and increased lung strength.

376.

Vitamin D supplementation protects children against respiratory infections

"Vitamin D supplementation significantly reduced the risk of acute respiratory infections in winter among Mongolian children with vitamin D deficiency."

Camargo CA Jr, Ganmaa D, et al. **Randomized trial of vitamin D supplementation and risk of acute respiratory infection in Mongolia.** *Pediatrics* 2012 Sep; 130(3): e561-67.

- During winter, 143 school children drank milk every day that was fortified with 300 IU of vitamin D. Another group of 247 school children (the control group) drank milk that was not fortified with vitamin D.
- At the end of the trial, children in the vitamin D group had higher median serum vitamin D levels (19 ng/mL vs 7 ng/mL) and significantly fewer acute respiratory infections than children in the control group (rate ratio, RR = 0.52).
- After adjusting for potential confounders, vitamin D supplementation still reduced by half the risk of acute respiratory infections (RR = 0.50).

377.

Linday LA, Shindledecker RD, et al. **Effect of daily cod liver oil and a multivitamin-mineral supplement with selenium on upper respiratory tract pediatric visits by young, inner-city, Latino children: randomized pediatric sites.** *Ann Otol Rhinol Laryngol* 2004 Nov; 113(11): 891-901.

"Use of these nutritional supplements...was associated with a decrease in upper respiratory tract pediatric visits over time."

- Children 6 months to 5 years of age were randomized into two groups. One group received daily supplementation with cod liver oil (high in vitamin D) and a multivitamin. The control group did not receive daily supplementation.
- In the months to follow, the supplementation group had a statistically significant reduction in pediatric visits for upper respiratory tract infections.

378.

Low serum vitamin D levels are associated with recent upper respiratory tract infections

"The results from our paper provide additional evidence from a large, diverse population of the inverse association between serum [vitamin D] level and respiratory tract infections. Vitamin D supplementation may reduce the incidence of upper respiratory tract infections and exacerbations of respiratory tract diseases."

Ginde AA, Mansbach JM, Camargo CA Jr. **Association between serum 25-hydroxyvitamin D level and upper respiratory tract infection in the Third National Health and Nutrition Examination Survey**. *Arch Intern Med* 2009 Feb 23; 169(4): 384-90.

- This study examined the link between serum vitamin D levels and recent upper respiratory tract infections in 18,883 people 12 years of age and older.

- Study participants were placed into one of three groups based on their serum 25-hydroxyvitamin D levels: a) below 10 ng/mL (<25 nmol/L), b) 10 to less than 30 ng/mL (25-74.9 nmol/L), and c) 30 ng/mL or higher (≥75 nmol/L).

- Individuals with serum vitamin D levels of less than 10 ng/ml were 55% more likely to have had a recent upper respiratory tract infection when compared to those with levels of 30 ng/mL or higher (OR = 1.55).

- Asthmatic participants with serum vitamin D levels below 10 ng/mL were 5.67 times more likely to have had a recent upper respiratory tract infection when compared to those with levels of 30 ng/mL or higher.

379.

Insufficient vitamin D in children increases the risk of an upper respiratory tract infection

"Lower serum 25-hydroxyvitamin D levels were associated with increased risk of laboratory-confirmed viral respiratory tract infections in children."

Science M, Maguire JL, et al. **Low serum 25-hydroxyvitamin D level and risk of upper respiratory tract infection in children and adolescents.** *Clin Infect Dis* 2013 Aug; 57(3): 392-97.

- The study sought to determine whether vitamin D serum levels are associated with laboratory-confirmed viral respiratory tract infections in children.

- At the start of the study, researchers measured the serum 25-hydroxyvitamin D levels of 743 children 3-15 years of age. The children were then followed during the respiratory virus season.

- A total of 229 children developed at least one laboratory-confirmed viral respiratory tract infection.

- Lower vitamin D levels and younger age were correlated with an increased risk of viral respiratory tract infections.

- Serum 25-hydroxyvitamin D levels that were less than 75 nmol/L significantly increased the risk of viral respiratory tract infections (hazard ratio, HR = 1.51). Levels below 50 nmol/L increased the risk by nearly 70% (HR = 1.67).

380.

Vitamin D protects children against acute lower respiratory infections

"Vitamin D supplementation is a low-cost, low-risk intervention that providers should consider for children, especially those at high risk for acute lower respiratory infection."

Larkin A, Lassetter J. **Vitamin d deficiency and acute lower respiratory infections in children younger than 5 years: identification and treatment.** *J Pediatr Health Care* 2014 Nov-Dec; 28(6): 572-82.

- Acute lower respiratory infection is a leading cause of childhood mortality.
- Thirteen studies found that vitamin D deficiency is associated with an increased risk or severity of acute lower respiratory infections.
- Vitamin D supplementation for children is recommended.

381.

Łuczyńska A, Logan C, et al. **Cord blood 25(OH)D levels and the subsequent risk of lower respiratory tract infections in early childhood: the Ulm birth cohort.** *Eur J Epidemiol* 2014 Aug; 29(8): 585-94.

"Our findings suggest that vitamin D deficiency at birth is associated with increased risk of lower respiratory tract infections. The association seems strongest in infants born in fall."

- Vitamin D levels were measured in the umbilical cord blood of 777 newborns.
- Newborns with vitamin D cord blood levels less than 25 nmol/L were significantly more likely to develop lower respiratory tract infections in the first year of life than newborns with levels above 50 nmol/L (RR = 1.32).

382.

Acute lower respiratory infections are much more severe in children with insufficient vitamin D

"Significantly more children admitted to the pediatric intensive care unit with acute lower respiratory infection were vitamin D deficient. These findings suggest that the immunomodulatory properties of vitamin D might influence acute lower respiratory infection disease severity."

McNally JD, Leis K, et al. **Vitamin D deficiency in young children with severe acute lower respiratory infection.** *Pediatr Pulmonol* 2009 Oct; 44(10): 981-88.

- The serum 25-hydroxyvitamin D levels of 95 young children hospitalized with acute lower respiratory infections were compared to 92 controls.
- Children with the most severe respiratory infections had significantly lower vitamin D levels than a) children with respiratory infections not requiring intensive care, and b) the control group without respiratory symptoms.

383.

Roth DE, Shah R, et al. **Vitamin D status and acute lower respiratory infection in early childhood in Sylhet, Bangladesh.** *Acta Paediatr* 2010 Mar; 99(3): 389-93.

"Acute lower respiratory tract infection is the most important global cause of childhood death. Vitamin D [deficiency] was associated with acute lower respiratory tract infection in a matched case control study."

- In this study, children 1 to18 months of age hospitalized with acute lower respiratory tract infection were matched to controls. The average vitamin D level among the sick children was significantly lower (29.1 nmol/L) when compared to the control group (39.1 nmol/L).
- For each 10 nmol/L increase in the serum vitamin D level, the likelihood of acute lower respiratory tract infection was decreased by half (OR = 0.53).

384.

Severe lower respiratory infections are significantly more likely to occur in children with a vitamin D deficiency

"Subclinical vitamin D deficiency and nonexclusive breastfeeding in the first 4 months of life were significant risk factors for severe acute lower respiratory infection."

Wayse V, Yousafzai A, et al. **Association of subclinical vitamin D deficiency with severe acute lower respiratory infection in Indian children under 5 y.** *Eur J Clin Nutr* 2004, 58: 563-67.

- This study compared children under 5 years of age who were diagnosed with severe acute lower respiratory infection (ALRI) to healthy controls to find out whether subclinical vitamin D deficiency increases the risk of ALRI.
- Children with severe ALRI were significantly less likely than controls to have serum 25-hydroxyvitamin D levels greater than 22.5 nmol/L (OR = 0.09). Exclusive breastfeeding in the first 4 months of life also significantly reduced the risk of developing ALRI (OR = 0.42).

385.

Inamo Y, Hasegawa M, et al. **Serum vitamin D concentrations and associated severity of acute lower respiratory tract infections in Japanese hospitalized children.** *Pediatr Int* 2011 Apr; 53(2): 199-201.

"Significantly more children with acute lower respiratory infection (ALRI) who needed supplementary oxygen and ventilator management were vitamin D deficient. These findings suggest that the immuno-modulatory properties of vitamin D may influence the severity of ALRI."

- This study investigated whether there is a link between vitamin D deficiency and the severity of respiratory infections in children hospitalized with ALRI.
- Children with ALRI and a vitamin D deficiency (less than 15 ng/mL) were significantly more likely to require oxygen and ventilator management.

386.

Medical doctors recommend vitamin D supplementation for healthcare workers as an alternative to influenza vaccination

"Some healthcare workers may be hesitant to take a vaccine because it contains a mercury preservative — thimerosal — which can be harmful to their health.... Because it has been well documented that a vitamin D deficiency can precipitate the influenza virus, we strongly recommend that all healthcare workers and patients be tested and treated for vitamin D deficiency to prevent exacerbation of a respiratory infection."

Edlich RF, Mason SS, et al. **Pandemic preparedness for swine flu influenza in the United States.** *J Environ Pathol Toxicol Oncol* 2009; 28(4): 261-64.

- This paper outlined strategies to limit the spread of influenza and urged healthcare workers and patients to be tested and treated for vitamin D deficiency.
- Vitamin D deficiency increases susceptibility to viral respiratory infections.
- Evidence was provided suggesting that optimal serum vitamin D levels to prevent deficiency are 50-75 ng/mL and the optimal dose of vitamin D for adults is 4,000 to 5,000 IU daily.

Non-Vaccination by Doctors and Nurses

Many pediatricians and family doctors do not vaccinate their own children in accordance with official recommendations. Some reject MMR, hepatitis B, Hib, pneumococcus, chickenpox, rotavirus, and/or influenza vaccines for their own children while others postpone MMR or pertussis until the child is older. In one study, 10% of general pediatricians and 21% of pediatric specialists admitted they do not plan to follow CDC guidelines in vaccinating their own children in the future. The most common reasons why physicians withhold vaccines for their own children are concerns about safety, the child's immune system is not ready, and too many vaccines are given at once.

Numerous studies confirm that healthcare workers throughout the world have low acceptance of vaccinations. For example, after three months of being told to vaccinate against pertussis, only 2% of Israeli nurses did so. In England, 57% of healthcare workers reject the seasonal influenza vaccine. In Italy, 70% of physicians and 89% of nurses reject influenza vaccines. In China, the influenza vaccine is rated as a second-class vaccine; just 21% of Chinese nurses and 13% of doctors are vaccinated against influenza.

For more than two decades, German guidelines urged healthcare workers to get vaccinated against influenza but only 39% of physicians and 17% of nurses receive a seasonal influenza vaccine. In Brazil, after health authorities ended a campaign encouraging healthcare workers to vaccinate against influenza, just 13% received an influenza vaccine.

The main reasons that healthcare workers are "noncompliant" and reject influenza vaccines include a) fear of side effects, b) they had serious adverse effects after previous vaccinations, c) belief that the vaccine will cause the disease, and d) little trust in its effectiveness. Many nurses also believe that parents have a right to decide whether to vaccinate their children. They demand this same respect for themselves.

387.

Pediatricians reject vaccines for their own children

"Ten percent of pediatricians and 21% of pediatric specialists claim they would not follow [CDC] recommendations for future progeny. Despite their education, physicians in this study expressed concern over the safety of vaccines."

Martin M, Badalyan V. **Vaccination practices among physicians and their children.** *OJPed* 2012 Sep; 2(3): 228-35.

- Researchers surveyed 582 pediatricians to determine whether they followed CDC guidelines in vaccinating their own children, and whether they plan to vaccinate their future children.

- Five percent of general pediatricians and 8% of subspecialist pediatricians (i.e., neonatologists, pediatric cardiologists) do not follow CDC vaccination guidelines.

- Ten percent of general pediatricians and 21% of subspecialist pediatricians planned to reject at least one vaccine for their future children.

- Despite increases in the incidence of measles, 5% of general pediatricians and 19% of subspecialist pediatricians planned to postpone MMR for their future children until after 18 months of age.

- A significant number of subspecialist pediatricians also planned to reject rotavirus (12%), meningococcal (9%) and hepatitis A (6%) vaccines for their future children.

- The most common reasons why pediatricians have already avoided at least one vaccine for their children, or plan to avoid vaccines for future children, are concerns about safety and too many vaccines given at once.

388.

Many pediatricians do not vaccinate their own children according to official recommendations

"A relatively large proportion of non-pediatric physicians do not follow, nor plan to follow, current immunization recommendations for their own children. Despite their scientific training and education, they express the same concerns as those that prevail in the public."

Posfay-Barbe KM, Heininger U, et al. **How do physicians immunize their own children? Differences among pediatricians and non-pediatricians.** *Pediatrics* 2005 Nov; 116(5): e623-33.

- Researchers surveyed 915 Swiss pediatricians and non-pediatric physicians (general practitioners and specialists) to determine how they vaccinated their own children, and how they would vaccinate them in the current year.

- Eight percent of pediatricians did not allow their own children to receive all of the officially recommended vaccines and 34% deviated from the officially recommended timing of vaccinations for their own children.

- Many pediatricians did not vaccinate their own children against hepatitis B (32%) or Hib (29%). Just 13% vaccinated their own children against influenza, 5% against pneumococcus, and 3% against varicella.

- Fourteen percent of non-pediatric physicians and 6 percent of pediatricians did not allow their own children to receive the first dose of MMR prior to 2 years of age, and 5% of non-pediatric physicians did not allow their own children to receive MMR at any age.

- Nine percent of non-pediatric physicians and 3 percent of pediatricians did not allow their own children to receive the first dose of a pertussis vaccine (DTP or DTaP) at the recommended age of 2 to 6 months.

- Some physicians rejected vaccines for their own children because they sought infection-driven rather than vaccine-induced immunity. The MMR vaccine was rejected because it was thought to be more harmful than the disease. Some vaccines were withheld due to concerns about safety and an immune overload.

389.

Pediatricians and family doctors do not recommend to parents that their children receive all vaccines

"We conclude that physician characteristics and concerns about childhood immunizations are associated with not recommending all childhood vaccines."

Gust D, Weber D, et al. **Physicians who do and do not recommend children get all vaccinations.** *J Health Commun* 2008 Sep; 13(6): 573-82.

- Researchers surveyed 250 pediatricians and 484 family practitioners who see at least five pediatric patients per week to determine whether they recommend to parents that children receive all available vaccines.
- Eleven percent of pediatricians and family doctors do not recommend to parents that their children should receive all vaccines.
- When compared with physicians who recommended all vaccines, family practitioners were significantly more likely than pediatricians to not recommend all vaccines for children (odds ratio, OR = 2.9) and to have concerns about the safety of childhood vaccination (OR = 2.0).

390.

Anastasi D, Di Giuseppe G, et al. **Paediatricians knowledge, attitudes, and practices regarding immunizations for infants in Italy.** *BMC Public Health* 2009 Dec 14; 9: 463.

- Researchers surveyed 156 Italian pediatricians to determine their knowledge, attitudes and behavior regarding vaccinations for infants.
- Just 10% of pediatricians had a very favorable attitude toward the utility of recommended vaccines for infants.
- Just 26% of pediatricians routinely administered recommended vaccines (which include measles, Hib and pertussis) to their patients.

391.

Pediatricians do not vaccinate their own children against chickenpox; doctors refuse vaccines for influenza, pertussis, and hepatitis B

"Many physicians voiced reservations about routine use of the varicella vaccine for healthy children."

Katz-Sidlow RJ, Sidlow R. **A look at the pediatrician as parent: experience with the introduction of varicella vaccine.** *Clin Pediatr (Phila)* 2003 Sep; 42(7): 635-40.

- Researchers surveyed 764 New York pediatricians to determine whether their choices in vaccinating their own children against chickenpox differed from their recommendations for their patients.

- Fifteen percent of surveyed pediatricians did not routinely recommend the chickenpox vaccine for their patients and 12% did not vaccinate their own eligible children against chickenpox.

392.

Pulcini C, Massin S, et al. **Factors associated with vaccination for hepatitis B, pertussis, seasonal and pandemic influenza among French general practitioners: a 2010 survey.** *Vaccine* 2013 Aug; 31(37): 3943-49.

- Researchers surveyed 1431 self-employed general practitioners (family doctors) in France to determine whether they received occupational vaccines.

- Twenty-three percent of general practitioners in France did not receive a seasonal influenza vaccine, 27% did not receive a hepatitis B vaccine, and 36% were not vaccinated against pertussis.

393.

Many European doctors think that measles is a harmless disease and do not recommend mandatory MMR vaccines

"Many general practitioners shared the common misconception that measles is not a serious health threat, even though half of them had encountered measles."

Pulcini C, Massin S, et al. **Knowledge, attitudes, beliefs and practices of general practitioners towards measles and MMR vaccination in south-eastern France in 2012.** *Clin Microbiol Infect* 2014 Jan; 20(1): 38-43.

- Researchers surveyed 329 general practitioners (GPs) in southeastern France to determine their attitudes toward measles and MMR vaccination.
- Eighty percent of GPs stated that most parents/patients consider measles a harmless disease.
- Thirty-three percent of GPs do not think that MMR vaccination should be mandatory for children under 2 years of age.
- Thirteen percent of GPs think that measles is a harmless disease and 12% are not convinced that a second dose of MMR is useful.
- Doctors who practiced alternative medicine were excluded from the study.

394.

Simone B, Carrillo-Santisteve P, Lopalco PL. **Healthcare workers' role in keeping MMR vaccination uptake high in Europe: a review of evidence.** *Euro Surveill* 2012 Jun 28; 17(26). pii: 20206.

- Researchers reviewed 28 European studies to determine the knowledge, attitudes and practices of health professionals toward measles/MMR vaccination and their influence on parental vaccination choices.
- Many European doctors do not recommend MMR for children.

395.

Israeli nurses reject pertussis and influenza vaccines

"In our study the nurses expressed an array of negative feelings against vaccines. These feelings include anger at the authorities, anger at loss of independence, fear of a new vaccine (being a guinea pig), fear of the side effects, and more. This is especially striking as their everyday routine work includes immunizing infants with this same pertussis vaccine."

Baron-Epel O, Bord S, et al. **What lies behind the low rates of vaccinations among nurses who treat infants?** *Vaccine* 2012 May 2; 30(21): 3151-54.

- Numerous studies confirm that healthcare workers all around the world have low acceptance of vaccinations.

- After three months of being told to vaccinate against pertussis, only 2% of Israeli nurses did so.

- The purpose of this study was to determine why nurses do not vaccinate themselves against pertussis even though they vaccinate infants against pertussis every day.

- The majority of nurses do not trust health authorities and have strong feelings against being told that they must be vaccinated.

- The nurses were concerned about side effects and believed that the risk of contracting the disease was not worth the risk of being injected. They felt this way toward both pertussis and influenza vaccines.

- The nurses also believe that parents have a right to decide whether to vaccinate their children. They demanded this same respect for themselves.

- The authors of this study believe that health authorities must convince nurses that they are unethical for refusing vaccines, and they need an increased perception of themselves as "transmitters of diseases."

396.

Doctors and nurses in Italy and England reject influenza vaccines

"Despite almost a decade of efforts, the vaccination coverage rates registered at our hospital steadily remain unsatisfactory.... During the last influenza season (2013/14), vaccination coverage rates by occupation type resulted in 30% among physicians, 11% among nurses and 9% among other clinical personnel."

Alicino C, Iudici R, et al. **Influenza vaccination among healthcare workers in Italy: the experience of a large tertiary acute-care teaching hospital.** *Hum Vaccin Immunother* 2015 Jan; 11(1): 95-100.

- Healthcare workers in Italy reject seasonal influenza vaccinations despite being subjected to a comprehensive multi-year, multi-faceted intervention project designed to increase vaccination rates.

397.

Head S, Atkin S, et al. **Vaccinating health care workers during an influenza pandemic.** *Occup Med (Lond)* 2012 Dec; 62(8): 651-54.

"During the 2009 pandemic, healthcare workers refused H1N1 vaccination due to concerns about clinical effectiveness, side effects and perceptions that H1N1 infection was not generally severe."

- Researchers surveyed healthcare workers in London during the 2009-10 H1N1 influenza pandemic to determine why so many refused vaccination.

- Forty-one percent of healthcare workers refused an H1N1 influenza vaccine and 57% rejected a seasonal influenza vaccine.

398.

Doctors and nurses in China and Spain reject influenza vaccines

"Annual influenza vaccination is recommended for health care workers in many countries. However, compliance rates with influenza vaccination are commonly low."

Seale H, Wang Q, et al. **Influenza vaccination amongst hospital health care workers in Beijing.** *Occup Med (Lond)* 2010 Aug; 60(5): 335-39.

- In Beijing, the influenza vaccine is rated as a "second-class vaccine."
- Only 21% of nurses and 13% of doctors were vaccinated against influenza.
- Forty percent of healthcare workers agree that "the flu vaccine can cause flu in some people."

399.

Vírseda S, Restrepo MA, et al. **Seasonal and Pandemic A (H1N1) 2009 influenza vaccination coverage and attitudes among healthcare workers in a Spanish University Hospital.** *Vaccine* 2010 Jul 5; 28(30): 4751-57.

"Influenza vaccination coverage among healthcare workers remains the lowest compared with other priority groups for immunization."

- During the 2009 influenza season, more than half of all healthcare workers in a Spanish hospital refused the seasonal influenza vaccine and only 16.5% received an H1N1 pandemic vaccine.
- Healthcare workers who refused the pandemic vaccine had "doubts about vaccine efficacy" and "fear of adverse reactions."

400.

Doctors and nurses in Germany and the USA reject influenza vaccines

"Acceptance of the influenza vaccination by medical personnel is low."

Wicker S, Rabenau HF, et al. **Influenza vaccination compliance among health care workers in a German university hospital.** *Infection* 2009 Jun; 37(3): 197-202.

- For more than two decades, German guidelines urged healthcare workers to get vaccinated against seasonal influenza yet influenza vaccination rates among doctors and nurses remain low.
- Just 39% of physicians and 17% of nurses receive a seasonal influenza vaccine.
- The main reasons that healthcare workers are "noncompliant" and reject influenza vaccines include fear of side effects, belief that the vaccine will cause the disease, and little trust in its effectiveness.

401.

Clark SJ, Cowan AE, Wortley PM. **Influenza vaccination attitudes and practices among US registered nurses.** *Am J Infect Control* 2009 Sep; 37(7): 551-56.

"Concerns about adverse reactions and vaccine effectiveness continue to be barriers to influenza vaccination among registered nurses."

- A survey of 1,017 U.S. registered nurses revealed that 41% did not receive an influenza vaccine during the previous influenza season.
- The most common reason for rejecting the influenza vaccine was concern about adverse reactions.

402.

Doctors and nurses in Canada and Brazil reject influenza vaccines

"Influenza vaccination among healthcare workers is poor."

Norton SP, Scheifele DW, et al. **Influenza vaccination in paediatric nurses: cross-sectional study of coverage, refusal, and factors in acceptance.** *Vaccine* 2008 Jun 2; 26(23): 2942-48.

- Many of the Canadian nurses that refused influenza vaccination did so because they believed it would not provide a personal benefit.

403.

Takayanagi IJ, Cardoso MR, et al. **Attitudes of health care workers to influenza vaccination: why are they not vaccinated?** *Am J Infect Control* 2007 Feb; 35(1): 56-61.

"Compliance rates with influenza vaccination among health care workers are historically low."

- Brazilian health authorities initiated a campaign encouraging healthcare workers to vaccinate against influenza, resulting in a compliance rate of 34%.

- When authorities ended their educational intervention, compliance rates dropped to 20% in the following year and just 13% in the year after that.

- Some of the top reasons given for rejecting influenza vaccination included a) risk of serious adverse effects, b) had serious adverse effects after previous vaccinations, and c) considered the vaccine to be ineffective or unnecessary.

404.

Doctors and nurses in many different countries resist influenza vaccines

"Numerous international vaccination programs have tried to encourage healthcare workers to be vaccinated but have met with surprising resistance."

Hofmann F, Ferracin C, et al. **Influenza vaccination of healthcare workers: a literature review of attitudes and beliefs.** *Infection* 2006 Jun; 34(3): 142-47.

- Top reasons many healthcare workers refuse the influenza vaccine are fear of adverse reactions and doubts about vaccine efficacy.

405.

Landelle C, Vanhems P, et al. **Influenza vaccination coverage among patients and healthcare workers in a university hospital during the 2006-2007 influenza season.** *Vaccine* 2012 Dec 17; 31(1): 23-26.

"Despite years of public health effort to increase vaccine uptake among populations recommended for influenza vaccination, immunization rates remain low among patients and healthcare workers."

406.

Hollmeyer HG, Hayden F, et al. **Influenza vaccination of health care workers in hospitals — a review of studies on attitudes and predictors.** *Vaccine* 2009 Jun 19; 27(30): 3935-44.

"Our findings indicate that if healthcare workers get immunized against influenza, they do so primarily for their own benefit and not for the benefit to their patients."

- Despite guidelines in many countries recommending influenza vaccination of healthcare workers to protect their patients, influenza vaccination rates among healthcare workers are universally low.

Education Level of Non-Vaccinating Parents

The studies in this chapter confirm that parents who don't vaccinate their children are highly educated, value scientific knowledge and are sophisticated at researching vaccines. Mothers with college degrees are the most likely to refuse vaccines for their children. Mothers who never graduated from high school are the most likely to fully vaccinate their children.

407.

Unvaccinated children come from families with highly educated mothers who don't let doctors influence their decisions

"Unvaccinated children tended to be white, to have a mother who was married and had a college degree, to live in a household with an annual income exceeding $75,000, and to have parents who expressed concerns regarding the safety of vaccines and indicated that medical doctors have little influence over vaccination decisions for their children."

Smith PJ, Chu SY, Barker LE. **Children who have received no vaccines: who are they and where do they live?** *Pediatrics* 2004; 114: 187-95.

- This study analyzed the vaccination histories of 151,720 children 19 to 35 months of age to determine whether unvaccinated children come from families with different characteristics than children who are under-vaccinated.

- Under-vaccinated children were significantly more likely to be black, to have a younger mother who was not married, to have completed fewer than 12 years of high school, and live in a household below the poverty level.

- Unvaccinated children were significantly more likely to be white, to have a mother who was at least 30 years old and married, to have a college degree, and live in a household with an annual income greater than $75,000.

- The parents of unvaccinated children were significantly more likely than the parents of under-vaccinated children to express concerns regarding vaccine safety (relative risk, RR = 17.0) and to say that doctors have no influence over vaccination decisions for their children (RR = 8.2).

- In the U.S. population of children 19 to 35 months of age, about 37% are under-vaccinated and just 0.3% are completely unvaccinated.

- Once parents have made a decision not to vaccinate, they are unlikely to be persuaded to change their mind.

408.

Mothers who don't vaccinate their children are highly educated, value scientific knowledge and are sophisticated at researching vaccines

"Low maternal educational levels and low socioeconomic status were associated with high [vaccination] completion rates. Also, completion rates were high in Hispanic and non-Hispanic Black families with low income-to-poverty ratios."

Kim SS, Frimpong JA, et al. **Effects of maternal and provider characteristics on up-to-date immunization status of children aged 19 to 35 months.** *Am J Public Health* 2007 Feb; 97(2): 259-66.

- The study analyzed national immunization data on 11,860 children 19 to 35 months of age to evaluate maternal characteristics that may be associated with whether the child is fully vaccinated.
- Mothers with college degrees and high incomes were the least likely to fully vaccinate their children. Mothers without a high school diploma, and poor minority families, were the most likely to fully vaccinate their children.

409.

Gullion JS, Henry L, Gullion G. **Deciding to opt out of childhood vaccination mandates.** *Public Health Nurs* 2008 Sep-Oct; 25(5): 401-8.

"Evidence of sophisticated data collection and information processing was a repeated theme in the interview data."

- This study investigated the attitudes and beliefs of parents who consciously choose not to vaccinate their children.
- Parents who did not vaccinate their children, a) value scientific knowledge, b) are sophisticated at collecting and processing information on vaccines to make their decisions, and c) show little trust in the medical community.

410.

Highly educated Israeli mothers are the most likely to refuse vaccines for their children

*"The ideological parents who don't [vaccinate their children] are very hard to persuade. But for parents who miss one or two vaccinations, there is room for intervention."**

Aharon AA, Nehama H, et al. **Reasons why parents do not comply with recommended pediatric vaccines.** Study presentation was made at the 5th International Jerusalem Conference on Health Policy, ICC Jerusalem Convention Center, June 3-5, 2013.

- This study analyzed the health records of 14,232 Israeli children 3 years of age to determine why some of them are not fully vaccinated and to evaluate maternal characteristics associated with non-vaccination.
- University-educated mothers were more than twice as likely to refuse vaccines compared to mothers with a high school education.
- Jewish and Christian parents were significantly more likely than Muslim parents to refuse vaccines for their children.
- Mothers with socioeconomic advantages were more likely to refuse vaccines due to their research and ideology, choosing which vaccines, if any, to permit.
- Poor mothers were more likely to miss vaccines because of behavioral or cultural blocks and lack of knowledge or organization.
- This study was conducted by the University of Haifa and funded by the Israel National Institute for Health Policy Research.

*This quote was provided by the author in an article — **More Israeli parents refusing to vaccinate their babies according to state regulations** — published in *Haaretz.com* 2013, June 4.

411.

Highly educated parents and healthcare workers reject vaccines for their children

"Determinants of a fully negative attitude [toward any new vaccine] were a high education of the parent [and] being a healthcare worker."

Hak E, Schönbeck Y, et al. **Negative attitude of highly educated parents and health care workers towards future vaccinations in the Dutch childhood vaccination program.** *Vaccine* 2005 May 2; 23(24): 3103-7.

- Researchers surveyed 283 Dutch parents to determine their attitudes toward future vaccines for their children against diseases such as influenza, pneumonia and hepatitis B.

- Eleven percent of Dutch parents had no intention of permitting their children to receive any new vaccine.

- Highly educated parents were 3 times more likely than other parents to reject new vaccines for their children (odds ratio, OR = 3.3). Healthcare workers were 4 times more likely to reject new vaccines for their children (OR = 4.2).

412.

Samad L, Tate AR, et al. **Differences in risk factors for partial and no immunisation in the first year of life: prospective cohort study.** *BMJ* 2006 Jun 3; 332(7553): 1312-13.

- Researchers surveyed 18,488 U.K. mothers when their infants were 9 months of age to compare maternal and demographic factors associated with non-vaccination, partial vaccination, and full vaccination.

- Mothers of non-vaccinated infants were older than mothers of fully vaccinated infants and significantly more educated (RR = 1.9).

- Mothers of partially vaccinated infants were significantly younger than mothers of fully vaccinated infants (rate ratio, RR = 1.7).

413.

Parents who exempt their children from vaccines are college-educated

"Parents requesting vaccination exemption in New Mexico tend to be White, non-Hispanic, and have at least a 4-year college degree."

New Mexico Department of Health, Office of the Secretary. **Department of health announces results of vaccination exemption survey.** *Press Release* 2013, November 18.

- This study surveyed 729 New Mexico parents who exempted their children from required vaccines to determine the demographics, attitudes and beliefs of this population.
- Sixty-seven percent of New Mexico parents who exempted their children from vaccines have at least a 4-year college degree; 74% are Anglo.

414.

O'Leary ST, Nelson C, Duran J. **Maternal characteristics and hospital policies as risk factors for nonreceipt of hepatitis B vaccine in the newborn nursery.** *Pediatr Infect Dis J* 2012 Jan; 31(1): 1-4.

"Maternal characteristics such as higher education and income are associated with nonreceipt of the hepatitis B vaccine during the perinatal period."

- Hospitals recommend that newborns receive a hepatitis B vaccine shortly after birth.
- Birth registry information on 64,425 newborns was matched with demographic data on their mothers to determine maternal characteristics associated with non-acceptance of hepatitis B vaccination.
- Mothers with a college master's degree are significantly less likely than mothers who have not graduated from high school to permit their newborns to receive a hepatitis B vaccine (odds ratio, OR = 1.66). They also have significantly higher incomes.

415.

Highly educated parents reject the MMR vaccine for their children

"Many parents make a conscious decision not to have their child immunized with MMR."

Pearce A, Law C, et al. **Factors associated with uptake of measles, mumps, and rubella vaccine (MMR) and use of single antigen vaccines in a contemporary UK cohort: prospective cohort study.** *BMJ* 2008 Apr 5; 336(7647): 754-57.

- Researchers surveyed 14,578 mothers to determine factors associated with not vaccinating their children with MMR by 3 years of age.

- Eleven percent of mothers did not vaccinate their children with MMR (6% of the children were unvaccinated against measles, mumps and rubella, while 5% received a measles-only vaccine).

- Children were significantly more likely to be unvaccinated with MMR or against measles if their mothers were highly educated (risk ratio, RR = 1.41).

- Mothers who rejected the MMR vaccine for their children but permitted them to receive a measles-only vaccine, were also highly educated (RR = 3.15).

- Parents who chose not to vaccinate their children with MMR voiced concerns about vaccine safety and did not trust the advice given by health professionals or the government.

416.

Highly educated parents are the least likely to allow their daughters to receive the HPV vaccine

"Further studies are needed to discover why, for example, parents with more education are less likely to agree to vaccination than parents with less education."

Ogilvie G, Anderson M, et al. **A population-based evaluation of a publicly funded, school-based HPV vaccine program in British Columbia, Canada: parental factors associated with HPV vaccine receipt.** *PLoS Med* 2010 May 4; 7(5): e1000270.

- This study surveyed 2,025 Canadian parents to determine factors associated with acceptance or rejection of the HPV vaccine for their daughters.
- Parents with higher levels of education were significantly more likely than less-educated parents to disallow the HPV vaccine for their daughters.
- Concern about HPV vaccine safety is the top reason that parents do not allow their daughters to receive the vaccine.

417.

Brewer NT, Fazekas KI. **Predictors of HPV vaccine acceptability: a theory-informed, systematic review.** *Prev Med* 2007 Aug-Sep; 45(2-3): 107-14.

"Parents with lower levels of education reported higher vaccine acceptability."

- This paper systematically reviewed 28 studies to determine parental beliefs regarding the human papilloma virus and factors associated with acceptance or rejection of the HPV vaccine for their daughters.
- Parents with higher levels of education were the least likely to accept the HPV vaccine for their daughters.

418.

College graduates reject HPV vaccination for their daughters; high school dropouts endorse it

"Subgroups more likely to endorse HPV vaccination included the less-than high-school.... Subgroups less likely to endorse vaccination were college graduates."

Constantine NA, Jerman P. **Acceptance of human papillomavirus vaccination among Californian parents of daughters: a representative statewide analysis.** *J Adolesc Health* 2007 Feb; 40(2): 108-115.

- This study surveyed 522 parents to determine factors that are associated with acceptance or rejection of HPV vaccination for their daughters.
- Parents who graduated from college were less likely to approve of HPV vaccination for their daughters. Parents without a high school degree were more likely to accept HPV vaccination.
- Asian-American parents were significantly less likely to accept HPV vaccination (OR = 0.44) while Hispanic parents were significantly more likely to allow their daughters to receive an HPV vaccine (OR = 2.12).
- Many of the parents who rejected HPV vaccination for their daughters were concerned about side effects.

419.

Rosenthal SL, Rupp R, et al. **Uptake of HPV vaccine: demographics, sexual history and values, parenting style, and vaccine attitudes.** *J Adolesc Health* 2008 Sep; 43(3): 239-45.

"Mothers who had less than a high school degree...were more likely to be favorable about their daughter being vaccinated."

- This study surveyed 153 mothers to determine parental factors that affect acceptance of HPV vaccination for their daughters.

Conflicts of Interest, False Studies, and Industry Control

The studies in this chapter provide strong evidence that biomedical research has been compromised by conflicts of interest, premeditated bias, and industry control. For example, in one study, 33% of scientists funded by the National Institutes of Health (NIH) admitted that they engaged in questionable scientific behavior during the previous 3 years. Nearly 16% of these top U.S. scientists changed the design, methodology or results of a study due to pressure from a funding source.

Conflicts of interest are pervasive within the vaccine industry and compromise the objectivity of vaccine safety research. For example, vaccine manufacturers sponsor research on their own products. Many authors of published papers on the safety of vaccines are paid consultants for or receive grant money from vaccine manufacturers. Medical journals rely on advertising revenue from pharmaceutical companies. Even the CDC receives money from the pharmaceutical industry that influences decisions it makes about the public welfare.

According to John Ioannidis, an expert on research bias, most published medical studies are false. Inaccurate findings can occur from a combination of factors, including the author's choice of study design, data, manipulation in the analysis or selective reporting of findings. Even large randomized studies with accurate research designs may provide false conclusions.

Oddly, there are no regulations guiding the composition of placebos nor is there a requirement to specify the composition of placebos in randomized, placebo-controlled trials published in journals. Placebos that are not neutral can influence study results. When studies do not provide sufficient details about placebo interventions, study replication is not possible.

Finally, anyone who questions the dominant views about vaccines is subject to threats, censorship, and loss of their livelihood. Doctors or scientists who question vaccines are considered threats to the public perception that all experts support vaccination. Proponents of vaccination suppress dissent in ways that are unfair. Methods include spreading rumors that threaten professional reputations, harassment, and denial of funding or access to research material. Suppression of dissent sends a warning to scientists and has a chilling effect on research. Free speech and the unimpeded ability to investigate unpopular topics are essential for scientific progress. In addition, authorities are tracking anti-vaccine tweets and are seeking efficient ways to censor anti-vaccine information on the internet.

420.

Many scientists intentionally fabricate data and falsify scientific research

"This is the first meta-analysis of surveys asking scientists about their experiences of misconduct. It found that, on average, about 2% of scientists admitted to have fabricated, falsified or modified data or results at least once and up to one third admitted a variety of other questionable research practices."

Fanelli D. **How many scientists fabricate and falsify research? A systematic review and meta-analysis of survey data.** *PloS One* 2009 May 29; 4(5): e5738.

- This study analyzed 21 surveys that asked scientists whether they have committed or know of a colleague who committed research misconduct that distorted scientific knowledge, including fabrication or falsification of data.

- Up to 5% (an average of 2%) of scientists admitted that they falsified, fabricated or modified data to improve results at least once. Up to 34% admitted that they engaged in other questionable research practices.

- Up to 33% (an average of 14%) of scientists had personal knowledge of colleagues who had falsified research data. Up to 72% knew about other questionable research practices committed by their colleagues.

- Some examples of questionable research practices included eliminating data points and altering the design, methodology or results of a study due to pressures from a funding source.

- Scientific misconduct may be more extensive in clinical, pharmacological and medical research than in other fields due to the large financial interests that foster substantial bias.

- In one survey, 81% of research trainees in the biomedical sciences were "willing to select, omit or fabricate data to win a grant or publish a paper."

- Because self-reports normally underestimate the true frequency of scientific misconduct, the findings in this paper may be conservative.

421.

Top scientists in the United States regularly engage in scientific misconduct that threatens the integrity of science

"Our findings reveal a range of questionable practices that are striking in their breadth and prevalence. U.S. scientists engage in a range of behaviors extending far beyond fabrication, falsification or plagiarism that can damage the integrity of science."

Martinson BC, Anderson MS, de Vries R. **Scientists behaving badly.** *Nature* 2005 Jun 9; 435: 737-38.

- Researchers surveyed 3,247 early- and mid-career U.S. scientists funded by the National Institutes of Health (NIH) and asked them to anonymously report their own scientific misbehavior during the previous three years.

- Overall, 33% of scientists funded by the NIH admitted that they engaged in questionable scientific behavior during the previous 3 years.

- Nearly 16% of NIH-funded scientists changed the design, methodology or results of a study due to pressure from a funding source; 15% dropped data points from analyses; 14% used inadequate or inappropriate research designs.

- Nearly 13% of NIH-funded scientists disregarded others' use of flawed data or questionable interpretation of data; 6% failed to present data that contradicted one's own previous research.

- Scientific misbehavior tended to increase as scientists gained in age and experience.

- Findings in this paper suggest that questionable scientific behavior that occurs on a regular basis may pose a greater threat to the integrity of scientific research than high-profile misconduct such as fraud.

- Estimates of scientific misbehavior found in this paper may be conservative.

422.

Scientists at top research institutions in the United States receive benefits from industry that compromise the integrity of their studies

"Our data demonstrate that senior-level investigators who responded to the survey receive a wide variety of industry-sponsored support which is important for their careers, and that industry support of research and researchers is pervasive in the clinical and research departments of top U.S. research institutions."

Tereskerz PM, Hamric AB, et al. **Prevalence of industry support and its relationship to research integrity.** *Account Res* 2009 Apr-Jun; 16(2): 78-105.

- An anonymous survey of 528 medical school faculty members at 33 top research institutions in the United States was conducted to learn how industry sponsorship influences scientific research.

- Two-thirds (67%) of medical researchers in this survey received some form of industry support, and 32% admitted that some portion of their salary was paid for by industry.

- Full professors were significantly more likely than associate professors to receive industry support, such as research grants, consulting agreements, royalty payments, joint commercial ventures, laboratory equipment, and various other financial arrangements.

- Of the respondents who received industry support for their research, 61% granted their industry sponsor prepublication review of manuscripts. Many also agreed to present results in a way that is favorable to the sponsor's product and to delay or completely withhold publication of results.

- A high percentage of respondents also reported that the interpretation of research data, the publication of research results, and scientific advancement in their field of research had all been compromised by industry support.

423.

The pharmaceutical industry has control of scientific journals, censors intellectual freedom, and threatens the integrity of biomedical research

"For a pharmaceutical company, delaying or minimizing knowledge of a side effect of a medication has cash value. Similarly, not publishing negative studies may shift the balance of subsequent meta-analyses."

Fava GA. **Preserving intellectual freedom in clinical medicine.** *Psychother Psychosom* 2009; 78: 1-5.

- This paper reviewed ways in which the pharmaceutical industry has gained control over many scientific societies and journals, censors intellectual freedom and threatens the integrity of biomedical research.

- Special interest groups representing pharmaceutical companies act as editors, reviewers and consultants to medical journals and research organizations, with the goal of systematically preventing the dissemination of information that conflicts with their interests.

- Pharmaceutical companies use the public relations industry to manipulate the interpretation of clinical trials with propaganda and to stifle dissent.

- The medical establishment is actively engaged in special interest advocacy that insulates the profession from intellectual freedom, alternative views and criticism of its prevailing practices.

424.

Medical journals benefit financially when they publish pharmaceutical industry studies that favor their products

"Journals have devolved into information laundering operations for the pharmaceutical industry."

Smith R. **Medical journals are an extension of the marketing arm of pharmaceutical companies.** *PLoS Med* 2005 May; 2(5): e138.

- This paper reviewed the evidence suggesting that medical journals and the pharmaceutical industry have a financially incestuous relationship that could compromise the integrity of science.

- Pharmaceutical companies provide medical journals with a substantial income from advertising. In addition, drug companies often purchase thousands of dollars worth of reprints if their papers are published. This creates a strong conflict of interest for journal editors and publishers.

- For a drug company, a favorable study published in a medical journal is immensely more valuable than ads.

- About 70% of clinical trials published in major journals are funded by the drug industry. Studies funded by the industry are 4 times more likely than studies funded from other sources to have findings favorable to the company.

- Drug companies have many ways to increase their odds of producing studies with favorable results. For example, they can suppress negative studies, conduct trials against inferior treatments, or show results that are most likely to impress, such as reduction in relative rather than absolute risk.

- The industry might also do subgroup analyses or use multiple endpoints or multi-location trials and select for publication those with favorable results.

- The peer-review process is defunct, inclined toward bias and abuse. Medical journals have become marketing tools of the drug industry, publishing studies that favor their products. Instead of publishing clinical trials, journals should consider critically describing them.

425.

Premeditated bias has infected the basic institutions and practices of the biomedical research community

"Today's biomedical researchers live in an organizational world within which lying and cheating are rife."

Noble JH. **Detecting bias in biomedical research: looking at study design and published findings is not enough.** *Monash Bioethics Review* 2007 Jan-Apr; 26(1-2): 24-45.

- Premeditated bias has infected the basic institutions and practices of the biomedical research community.
- Biomedical researchers and their sponsors publish skewed and misleading research findings.
- More than 65,000 product liability lawsuits have been filed against pharmaceutical drug manufacturers, which suggests that they and the FDA consider patient safety a low priority.
- This paper reviewed the technical means by which biomedical researchers produce studies that contain premeditated bias — fabricated data is just an extreme form — and makes recommendations on ways to counteract it.

426.

Glick JL. **Scientific data audit—a key management tool.** *Accountability in Research* 1992; 2(3): 153-68.

- Data audits by the Food and Drug Administration (FDA) found that 10-20% of studies contained misrepresented data, inaccurate reporting and fabricated experimental results.
- These findings resulted in 2% of clinical researchers being judged guilty of serious scientific misconduct.

427.

Conflicts of interest are pervasive within the vaccine industry and compromise the objectivity of vaccine safety research

"Vaccine manufacturers have financial motives and public health officials have bureaucratic reasons that might lead them to sponsor research that concludes vaccines are safe."

DeLong G. **Conflicts of interest in vaccine safety research.** *Account Res* 2012; 19(2): 65-88.

- This paper summarizes conflicts of interest that pervade the vaccine industry and offers suggestions on possible remedies.

- Vaccine manufacturers sponsor research on their own products.

- Many authors of published papers assessing the safety of vaccines are paid consultants for or receive grant money from vaccine manufacturers.

- Medical journals rely on advertising revenue from pharmaceutical companies.

- The vaccine industry employs three lobbyists for every member of Congress. Many lobbyists within the pharmaceutical industry were former members of Congress.

- The FDA and CDC may be reluctant to sponsor research that reveals safety problems associated with vaccines that they licensed and promoted because it could damage their reputations and reduce public trust.

- Reports of vaccine injury are not adequately investigated.

- Agencies that oversee vaccine safety should be prohibited from promoting vaccines.

- Data in vaccine safety studies should be released to the public so that independent scientists can replicate the findings.

428.

Authors of important studies published in top medical journals have conflicts of interest that influence study results

"Conflict of interest is widespread among the authors of published manuscripts and these authors are more likely to present positive findings."

Friedman LS, Richter ED. **Relationship between conflicts of interest and research results.** *J Gen Intern Med* 2004 Jan; 19(1): 51-56.

- Researchers analyzed 398 studies published in the top 2 medical journals — *New England Journal of Medicine* (NEJM) and *Journal of the American Medical Association* (JAMA) — to determine a) their sources of funding and b) whether there is a link between study findings and conflicts of interest.

- Private corporations funded 38% of the studies published in NEJM and 35% of the studies in JAMA. The top 5 companies sponsoring these studies were all large vaccine/drug manufacturers.

- Nearly 39% of the studies investigating pharmaceutical treatments had authors with conflicts of interest.

- There was a statistically significant relationship between studies that were conducted by authors with conflicts of interest and positive research findings (odds ratio, OR = 2.64). The association was even stronger when using a less restrictive conflict of interest definition: (OR = 7.32).

- The odds are extremely small that negative study results would be published by authors with conflicts of interest: (OR = 0.05).

- Authors with conflicts of interest are up to 20 times less likely to publish studies with negative findings than authors without conflicts of interest.

- This study provides strong evidence that conflicts of interest in biomedical research are pervasive and that current systems of oversight are ineffective at monitoring this serious threat to the integrity of science.

429.

Meta-analyses of pharmaceutical products do not report conflicts of interest

"Among a group of meta-analyses of pharmacological treatments published in high-impact biomedical journals, information concerning primary study funding and author conflicts of interest for the included randomized controlled trials were only rarely reported."

Roseman M, Milette K, et al. **Reporting of conflicts of interest in meta-analyses of trials of pharmacological treatments.** *JAMA* 2011 Mar 9; 305(10): 1008-17.

- Meta-analysis is a large study that uses statistical techniques to integrate data from several independent randomized controlled trials.
- This study investigated whether meta-analyses of pharmaceutical treatments report conflicts of interest disclosed in the original studies.
- Of 29 meta-analyses reviewed (which included 509 randomized, controlled studies) only 2 (7%) reported who funded the study and none reported the authors' financial ties with the pharmaceutical industry.
- In 7 of the 29 meta-analyses reviewed, every underlying study was funded by the pharmaceutical industry or had authors with financial ties to the drug industry. Yet, only 1 of these 7 meta-analyses reported the source of funding and none reported a monetary link between study authors and the industry.

430.

Roseman M, Turner EH, et al. **Reporting of conflicts of interest from drug trials in Cochrane reviews: cross sectional study.** *BMJ* 2012 Aug 16; 345: e5155.

"This study found that most Cochrane reviews of drug trials did not report information on trial funding sources or trial author-industry financial ties, including employment, from included trials. When this information was reported, patterns of reporting were inconsistent."

431.

The CDC receives money from the pharmaceutical industry that influences decisions it makes about the public welfare

"The CDC's image as an independent watchdog over the public health has given it enormous prestige, and its recommendations are occasionally enforced by law. Despite the agency's disclaimer, the CDC does receive millions of dollars in industry gifts and funding, both directly and indirectly, and several recent CDC actions and recommendations have raised questions about the science it cites, the clinical guidelines it promotes, and the money it is taking."

Lenzer J. **Centers for Disease Control and Prevention: protecting the private good?** *BMJ* 2015 May 15; 350: h2362.

- The CDC claims that it has no financial dealings with the manufacturers of commercial products but this is not true.
- In 1992, Congress passed legislation that created the non-profit CDC Foundation to encourage relationships between the CDC and industry. Pharmaceutical companies donate to the CDC Foundation.
- The CDC receives millions of dollars annually in "conditional funding" from corporations and the CDC Foundation. The CDC uses conditional funds to oversee controversial recommendations and studies. Corporations can punish the CDC if it conducts research that affects their profits.
- Industry funding inserts bias into treatment recommendations and study results which is unacceptable for a public health agency.
- The CDC has a systemic lack of oversight of its ethics program.
- The CDC's high credibility among physicians would be threatened if they learned that it takes money from pharmaceutical companies.
- The fact that the CDC takes money from industry cannot be fixed by asking the CDC to be more ethical and avoid conflicts of interest. U.S. legislators caused this problem and can make new laws to fix the problem.

432.

There is no requirement that the authors of prominent highly-cited randomized, placebo-controlled studies disclose composition of the placebo

"Failure to report placebo composition compromises the foundation on which medical decisions are based, and on which the fate of lives may rest."

Golomb BA, Erickson LC, et al. **What's in placebos: who knows? Analysis of randomized, controlled trials**. *Ann Intern Med* 2010; 153(8): 532-35.

- Although placebos can influence study results, there are no regulations guiding placebo composition.

- This study was designed to assess how often researchers specify the composition of placebos in randomized, placebo-controlled trials published in journals with a high impact factor. A total of 176 studies that used pills, injections and other treatment methods were included.

- In studies that used pills, 92% did not disclose placebo ingredients. In 74% of studies that used injections and 72% using other treatment methods, placebo composition was not disclosed.

- Placebos are widely believed to be physiologically inert. However, no substances are known to be physiologically inert.

- Placebos that are not neutral can have effects that influence study results.

- When studies do not provide sufficient details about placebo interventions, study replication is not possible.

- Studies that fail to identify placebo ingredients violate basic scientific standards.

433.

Most published medical studies are false

"For most study designs and settings, it is more likely for a research claim to be false than true. Moreover, for many current scientific fields, claimed research findings may often be simply accurate measures of the prevailing bias."

Ioannidis JP. **Why most published research findings are false.** *PloS Med* 2005 Aug; 2(8): e124.

- This paper demonstrates that most published research findings are false.
- Bias, which produces false findings, can occur from a combination of factors, including the authors' choice of study design, data, manipulation in the analysis or selective reporting of findings.
- Findings are less likely to be true when the effect is small, when there is great flexibility in the study design and analytical methods, when there are financial interests, and when more teams are seeking statistical significance.
- Some findings will be false due to chance variability despite an ideal study design, data, analysis and presentation.
- Even with large randomized studies and accurate research designs, bias is a major problem with manipulated analyses, outcomes and selective reporting.
- Data can be used inefficiently, researchers may fail to notice statistically significant relationships, or there could be conflicts of interest that ignore or hide significant findings.
- Conflicts of interest in biomedical research are common and rarely reported.
- Most biomedical research has a very low probability of providing true findings. Even large epidemiological studies may provide false conclusions.
- The peer-review process may be used to suppress the publication of findings that refute reviewers' existing beliefs in a scientific theory or their own findings. This can condemn an entire research field to false dogma.

434.

Highly-cited medical studies, even randomized controlled studies, are often refuted by subsequent studies

"Contradiction and initially stronger effects are not unusual in highly cited research of clinical interventions and their outcomes. Controversies are most common with highly cited non-randomized studies, but even the most highly cited randomized trials may be challenged and refuted over time."

Ioannidis JP. **Contradicted and initially stronger effects in highly cited clinical research.** *JAMA* 2005 Jul 13; 294(2): 218-28.

- Published studies on the efficacy of medical interventions are sometimes refuted by subsequent studies that either give opposite conclusions or show that the original findings were too strong.

- This paper compared 45 of the most highly cited studies against subsequent studies of comparable sample size and similar or better controlled designs. (The most highly cited studies receive the most attention and have the greatest influence over scientific thinking and debate.)

- Thirty-one percent of highly-cited original clinical research studies were either contradicted or shown to have exaggerated effects by subsequent studies.

- Eighty-three percent of highly-cited non-randomized studies, and 23% of randomized controlled studies, were either contradicted or shown to have exaggerated effects by subsequent studies.

- Studies that were not so highly cited had similar proportions of contradicted results as the highly cited ones.

- Publication bias, where journals favor the rapid and prominent publication of studies with statistically significant findings (versus those with no significant findings), may contribute to the high number of refuted studies.

- Findings from recent studies — even those with impressive evidence — should be read with caution.

435.

Anyone who is critical of vaccines may be unfairly suppressed, exposed to threats, censorship, and loss of their livelihood

"According to the highest ideals of science, ideas should be judged on their merits, and addressed through mustering evidence and logic. Suppression of dissent is a violation of these ideals."

Martin B. **On the Suppression of Vaccination Dissent.** *Sci Eng Ethics* 2015; 21(1): 143-57.

- Some proponents of vaccination believe that anyone who is critical of vaccines cannot be credible. They may be labeled anti-vaccine or anti-science, implying that there are no legitimate scientific concerns about vaccination.

- Doctors or scientists who question vaccines are considered threats to the public perception that all experts support vaccination.

- Anyone who questions the dominant views about vaccines is subject to abuse, including threats, formal complaints, censorship, and loss of their livelihood.

- Proponents of vaccination suppress dissent in ways that are unfair. Methods include spreading rumors that threaten professional reputations, harassment, and denial of funding or access to research material.

- There is a double standard in biomedical and vaccine research. When orthodox views are promoted, serious ethical violations such as undeclared conflicts of interest, using false placebos and withholding evidence, are often ignored.

- Suppression of dissent impedes open debate and deters vaccine supporters from considering all available evidence.

- Scientific advancement requires challenging orthodox ideas. Suppression of dissent sends a warning to scientists and has a chilling effect on research.

- Free speech and the unimpeded ability to investigate unpopular topics are essential for scientific progress.

436.

Authorities are tracking anti-vaccine information on the internet

"Information about social connections may be useful in the surveillance of opinions for public health purposes."

Zhou X, Coiera E, et al. **Using social connection information to improve opinion mining: identifying negative sentiment about HPV vaccines on Twitter.** *Stud Health Technol Inform* 2015; 216: 761-765.

- In this paper, researchers examined ways in which computer programs could be designed to improve surveillance methods on Twitter to more accurately identify anti-vaccine opinions.

437.

Dunn AG, Leask J, et al. **Associations between exposure to and expression of negative opinions about human papillomavirus vaccines on social media: an observational study.** *J Med Internet Res* 2015 Jun 10; 17(6): e144.

"This research may be useful for identifying individuals and groups currently at risk of disproportionate exposure to misinformation about HPV vaccines."

- In this paper, researchers sought to determine whether exposure to negative opinions about HPV vaccines on Twitter is associated with the subsequent expression of negative opinions.

- Between October 2013 and April 2014, 83,551 tweets that included terms related to HPV vaccines were analyzed by a "machine learning classifier" and classified as either negative or neutral/positive.

- Approximately 38% of people who were exposed to a majority of negative tweets about HPV vaccines subsequently posted a negative tweet, compared to 11% of people who were exposed to a majority of positive and neutral tweets (relative risk, RR = 3.46).

438.

Authorities want to censor free speech and anti-vaccine information on the internet

"Online communities with greater freedom of speech lead to a dominance of anti-vaccine voices. Moderation of content by editors can offer balance between free expression and factual accuracy. Health communicators and medical institutions need to step up their activity on the internet."

Venkatraman A, Garg N, Kumar N. **Greater freedom of speech on Web 2.0 correlates with dominance of views linking vaccines to autism.** *Vaccine* 2015 Mar 17; 33(12): 1422-25.

- In this paper, four large internet websites were analyzed to determine how much freedom of speech each site permits, as measured by viewpoints that support a link between vaccines and autism.

- YouTube allows users to search by relevance, which allows anyone's uploaded material to rise to the top of search results. Google's search algorithm gives advantage to web pages that have been linked to by many other web pages.

- Wikipedia has editors who remove information that is not supported by what they determine are reliable sources. PubMed only allows indexed scientific publications to show up in a search.

- In this study, anti-vaccine views were found to be more prevalent on websites where greater freedom of speech is permitted.

- With the rise of the internet, reliable and credentialed sources of information are not valued like they once were, which has allowed the vaccine-autism controversy to flourish.

- Changing Google's search algorithm to give advantage to "quality" sources could reduce anti-scientific views, but would not be as effective as moderation by human editors.

- In scientific situations, it may be desirable to block out dissenting opinions. Editors can modulate free speech to reduce alarmist vaccine viewpoints.

Index

D

N

Q

R

About the Author

Neil Z. Miller is a medical research journalist and Director of the *Thinktwice Global Vaccine Institute*. He has devoted the past 25 years to educating parents and health practitioners about vaccines, encouraging informed consent and non-mandatory laws. He is the author of several books on vaccines, including *Vaccine Safety Manual for Concerned Families and Health Practitioners, Make an Informed Vaccine Decision for the Health of Your Child* (with Dr. Mayer Eisenstein) and *Vaccines: Are They Really Safe and Effective?* Past organizations that he has lectured for include the International Chiropractic Pediatric Association, the International College of Integrative Medicine, Autism One, Maximized Living, and the Culture of Life Institute. Mr. Miller has a degree in psychology and is a member of Mensa. He lives in Northern New Mexico.

Purchasing Information

Miller's Review of Critical Vaccine Studies (ISBN: 978-188121740-4) may be purchased directly from *New Atlantean Press*. Call 505-983-1856. Or send $21.95 (in U.S. funds), plus $5.00 for media mail shipping (or $7.00 for priority shipping) to:

New Atlantean Press
PO Box 9638, Santa Fe, NM 87504
505-983-1856 (Telephone & Fax)
Email: think@thinktwice.com

This book is also available at many fine bookstores.

Bookstores/Libraries/Retail Buyers: Order from Midpoint Trade Books, Ingram, Baker &Taylor, or New Atlantean Press.

Parents, Chiropractors, Naturopaths, and other Non-Storefront Buyers: Take a 40% discount with the purchase of 5 or more copies (multiply the total cost of purchases x .60). Please add 9% for shipping. *Larger discounts are available.* Call or email us for case quantity discounts and shipping rates.

Shipping Rates

United States (1 or 2 books): Please add $5.00 for media mail (allow 1-3 weeks for your order to arrive) or include $2.00 extra ($7.00 total) for Priority shipping.
Canada and Mexico: Please add $24.00 for Global Priority shipping.
Europe, Asia and Australia: Please add $26.00 for Global Priority shipping.

More Vaccine Resources

Vaccine Safety Manual for Concerned Families and Health Practitioners, 2nd Edition (ISBN: 978-18812174037-4). The most extensive guide to vaccine-related diseases and vaccine risks. Includes more than 1,000 scientific citations. More than 100 charts, graphs and illustrations supplement the text. This encyclopedic health manual is an important addition to every family's home library and will be referred to again and again. Code: VSM (352 pages) $19.95.

Make an Informed Vaccine Decision (ISBN: 978-188121736-7). An excellent vaccine resource by Dr. Mayer Eisenstein, MD and Neil Z. Miller. Includes essential information on every childhood vaccine. Code: MIV (224 pages) $14.95.

Vaccines: Are They *Really* Safe and Effective? (ISBN: 978-188121730-5). An excellent introductory book on vaccine safety and efficacy issues. Includes 30 charts and more than 900 citations. Code: VAC (128 pages) $12.95.

ONLINE CATALOG: *New Atlantean Press* offers additional books and other resources:

www.vacbook.com / www.thinkchoice.com